S0-AKD-866

DIET AND OBESITY

DIET AND OBESITY

Edited by
George A. Bray, Jacques LeBlanc,
Shuji Inoue, and Masashige Suzuki

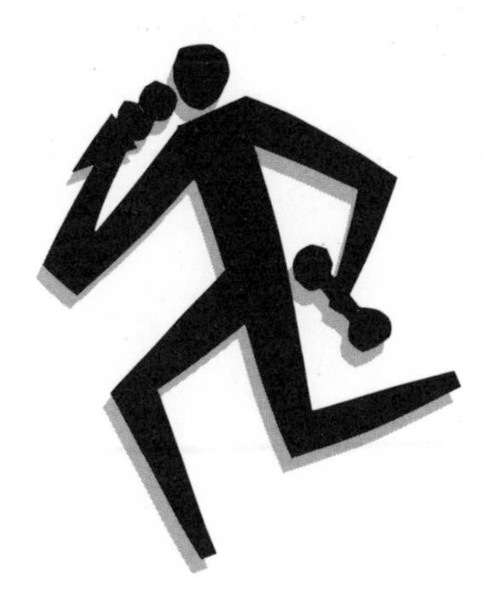

JAPAN SCIENTIFIC SOCIETIES PRESS
KARGER

Published jointly by
JAPAN SCIENTIFIC SOCIETIES PRESS
Hongo 6-2-10, Bunkyo-ku, Tokyo 113, Japan
ISBN 4-7622-2572-X
and
S. KARGER AG
P.O.Box, CH-4009 Basel, Switzerland
ISBN 3-8055-4980-6

Sole distribution rights outside Japan granted to S. KARGER AG, Basel.

Printed in Japan

Preface

Obesity is one of the most intensive health concerns of people in industrialized countries. Excess body fat deposition easily develops as the result of a positive energy balance. However, recent scientific evidence has indicated that several dietary and metabolic factors can enhance this unnecessay body fat deposition without excess energy intake. International Symposium on The Dietry and Metabolic Basis for Obesity and Its Prevention in Kyoto, October 29–30, 1987 was held to assess the factors of food, eating habits and exercise in modern-day living as they affect obesity. This book offers edited information presented at that meeting and, it is hoped, will further an understanding of dieting among nutritionists, of obesity among research scientists, and of appropriate food production for weight control among concerned industries.

Our thanks are extended to Hayashibara Biochemical Laboratories, Inc. and Towa Chemical Industry Co., Ltd. who sponsored the Symposium and the publication of this book.

August 1988

G.A. Bray
J. LeBlanc
S. Inoue
M. Suzuki

INTRODUCTION

Obesity and Alteration of Food Habits with Westernization

MASASHIGE SUZUKI*[1] AND NORIMASA HOSOYA*[2]

Biochemistry of Exercise and Nutrition, Institute of Health and Sport Sciences, The University of Tsukuba, Tsukuba 305,[1] *and Kokusai-Gakuin Saitama Junior College, Owmiya, Saitama 330,*[2] *Japan*

Obesity is the accumulation of excess body fat. This obviously occurs when energy intake exceeds energy expenditure. Such an energy imbalance is the result of overeating, under-exercising, a combination of the two, or a genetic or acquired defect in metabolism.

The characterized metabolic figures observed in the organisms accumulating excess body fat are stimulated lipogenesis in the liver and adipose tissue, hyper-triacylglycerolemia, increased lipoprotein lipase activity in the adipose tissue and the enhanced uptake and storing of circulating triacylglycerols by the adipose tissue. A decrease in diet-induced thermogenesis, the so-called energy futile system, is also observed in the obese (*1*). These metabolic and thermogenic alterations in the obese are mediated in common by insulin action. On the other hand, from an energy economy point of view, it has been suggested that dietary fat is stored in body fat more efficiently than dietary carbohydrate (*2*). Simply stated, when taken in excess, fat seems to be more fattening than carbohydrate.

The modernized food habits listed below seem to accelerate the

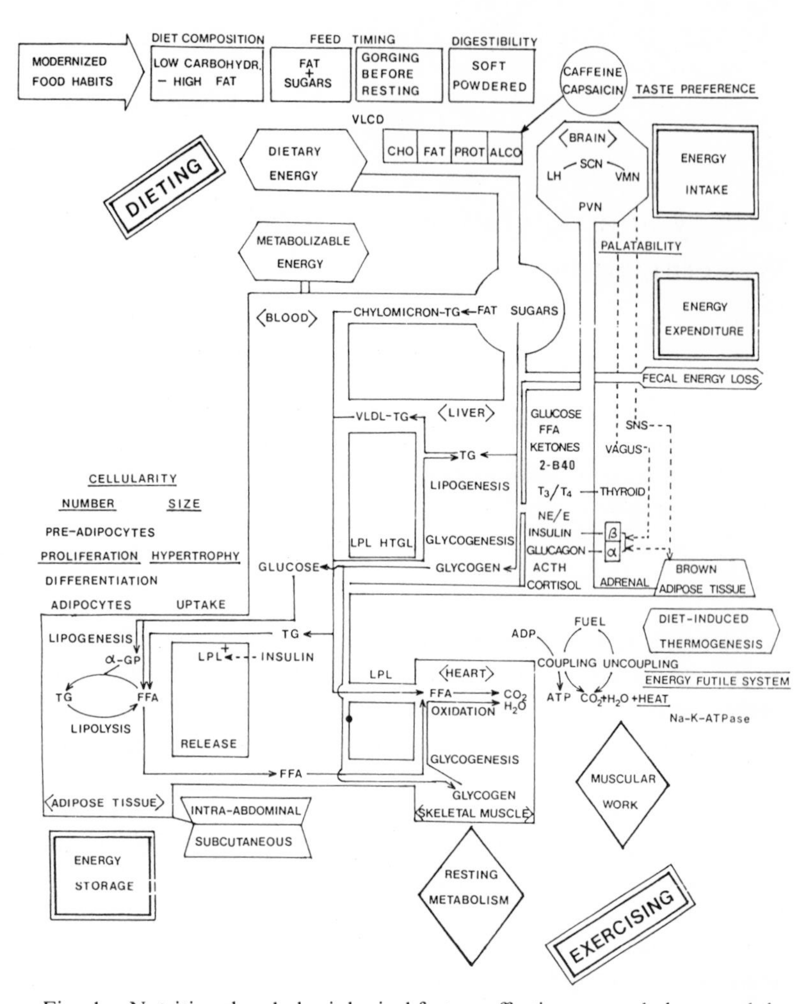

Fig. 1. Nutritional and physiological factors affecting energy balance and the development of obesity. VLCD, very-low calorie diet; LH, lateral hypothalamic area; SCN, suprachiasmatic nucleus; VMN, ventromedial nucleus; PVN, paraventricular nucleus; SNS, sympathetic nervous system; FFA, free fatty acids; 2-B40, 2-buten-4-olide; TG, triglycerides; VLDL, very-low density lipoproteins; LPL, lipoprotein lipase; HTGL, hepatic triglyceride lipase.

storage of ingested energy as body fat by nature regardless of the amount of energy ingested :

1) The decreased carbohydrate and increased fat proportions in daily energy intake (the increased energy density of foods and meals)

2) Gorging just before resting

3) The increase in simultaneous intake of fat and sugars

4) The increased consumption of cereals in powdered form rather than in grain form

5) The increased consumption of soft and digestible foods rather than hard and more difficult to digest foods

6) The increased consumption of alcohol

7) Others

These could also influence the regulation of energy intake. Therefore, in consideration of the characteristics of modern food habits, deeper understanding is needed through reviews and discussions of the biological systems regulating energy intake, expenditure and storage, and the effects of diet and exercise. Figure 1 indicates biochemical, physiological, and nutritional points to be discussed. By revealing the factors in modern individuals which allow unnecessary body fat accumulation without excess energy intake, this Symposium is expected to provide useful scientific information on foods, eating habits and exercise to prevent obesity.

REFERENCES

1. Girardier, L. and Stock, M. J. (1983). "Mammalian Thermogenesis," pp. 1-359. Chapman and Hall, London.
2. Danforth, E., Jr. (1985). Diet and obesity. *Am. J. Clin. Nutr.* **41**, 1132-1145.

Contents

Prevention of Excess Body Fat Deposition by Dieting and Exercise

DIETARY AND METABOLIC BASIS FOR EXCESS BODY FAT DEPOSITION

Diet and Obesity, Bray, G.A. et al., eds., pp. 3-15.
Japan Sci. Soc. Press, Tokyo/S. Karger, Basel (1988)

Regulation of Alimentation by Sugar Acids in Body Fluids

YUTAKA OOMURA,*[1],*[4] AKIRA NIIJIMA,*[2] AND ITSURO MATSUMOTO*[3]

Department of Physiology, Faculty of Medicine, Kyushu University, 60, Fukuoka 812,[1] Department of Physiology, Faculty of Medicine, Niigata University, Niigata 951,*[2] and Department of Physiology, Faculty of Medicine, Nagasaki Univerisity, Nagasaki 852,*[3] Japan*

Certain neurons are described as glucoreceptor neurons (GRN) if their activity increases dose dependently upon direct exposure to glucose. Other neurons are described as glucose-sensitive (GSN) if their spontaneous activity is diminished by direct exposure to glucose. GSNs can now be found in many discrete, identifiable neuronal centers although they are apparently most dense in the lateral hypothalamic area (LHA); GRNs in a similar way are probably most dense in the ventromedial nucleus of the hypothalamus (VMH). GSNs in the LHA and GRNs in the VMH were first actually described in 1969 (*1*) after J. Mayer suggested in 1955 that glucose-responsive neurons that might monitor blood glucose levels might be found there.

Glucoreceptor and glucose-sensitive are terms given to these neurons as a result of concepts that were accepted at the time of their discovery. These neurons are, in fact, not specific to glucose but

*[4]Present address: Toyama Medical and Pharmaceutical University, Toyama and Institute of Bio-Active Science, Nippon Zoki Pharmaceutical Co., Ltd., Yashiro-cho, Hyogo 673-14, Japan.

respond to most of the metabolites and hormones that have been found to either control feeding behavior or change in level with result of feeding.

Insulin, glucagon, calcitonin, and other endogenous factors affect both GRN and GSN in ways that depend on the state of satiation and the combination of factors present (*2*). The responses of these neurons to metabolites such as free fatty acids are consistent with the physiological levels of the respective substances at different times in the diurnal and feeding cycles. If these neurons were discovered today, with our present knowledge of their other properties, GSNs would probably be described as feeding control or hunger-related neurons and GRNs would be satiation control or satiety-related neurons.

I. ENDOGENOUS SUGAR ACIDS

Recently, a group of sugar acids has been found in the blood of rats. One of these recently identified metabolites induces feeding, and two others potently suppress feeding. The sugar acid 2(s), 4(s), 5-trihydroxypentanoic acid γ-lactone (2,4,5-TP) induces feeding, and 3(s), 4-dihydroxybutanoic acid γ-lactone (3,4-DB) and 2-buten-4-olide(2-B4O) suppress feeding (*3, 4*). The action of all three of these substances is mediated by GSNs and GRNs in the hypothalamus and medulla. These three substances were selected from among 18 that were measured in the blood by gas mass spectrometry. All 18 of the substances changed during food deprivation, but these three changed in ways that suggested the possibility of their affecting feeding behavior. Changes in the concentration of these three substances in blood during the time course of food deprivation are shown in Fig. 1 (*5*). During deprivation the level of 2,4,5-TP increased from 220 μM to a peak of about 360 μM at 12 hr, decreased slightly after 24 hr, then started to rise again and was still rising at 60 hr. The level of 3,4-DB increased from an initial level of about 120 μM to a peak of about 160 μM at 48 hr after the start of deprivation. The level of 2-B4O increased from an initial level of 3.5 μM up to 13.5 μM at 48–60 hr in a similar manner to 3,4-DB.

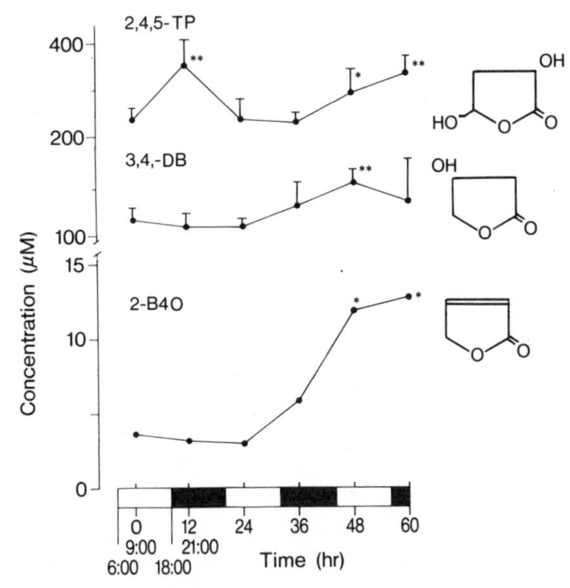

Fig. 1. Changes in 2,4,5-TP, 3,4-DB, and 2-B4O levels after food deprivation. 2,4,5-TP increased initially at normal feeding time and again after 2 days of deprivation, suggesting induction of drive to eat. 3,4-DB and 2-B4O increased in period of severe deprivation, which might be accounted for by starvation-induced anorexia. Although the absolute level of 2-B4O was far below those of 3,4-DB and 2,4,5-TP, its apparent sensitivity to deprivation was much greater. Abscissa, time: upper scale, hours of deprivation; lower scale, real time; black area, dark period. Ordinates, μM concentrations in rat plasma; note scale differences. Significantly different from basal level (*5*).

In agreement with the time courses of the changes, 2,4,5-TP increases and 3,4-DB depresses feeding, although the effects of both depended on the time of application, and the effects of 3,4-DB also depend on the route of application (*3*). When 2,4,5-TP was injected into the third cerebral ventricle at 1030, a dose of 2.5 μmol transiently induced feeding, but the total daily increase was not significant. Injection at 1900 increased food intake significantly until 2300 but not after. Injection intravenously or intraperitoneally at 1900 increased food consumption dose dependently, ranging from 17% for 100 μmol to 39% for 500 μmol. Injection of 2.5 μmol 3,4-DB into the third cerebral ventricle at 1630 significantly decreased food consumption for 12 hr and this recovered after 24 hr. Motor activity was not affected, and there was no other overt evidence of toxicity. Similar results were observed in rats deprived for 72 hr. Despite the effectiveness of injections into the third ventricle, injection of 100–500 μmol 3,4-DB intravenously or intraperitoneally at 1900 did not affect food consumption. The results of peripheral injections were attributed to either failure to cross the blood-brain barrier or adhesion of 3,4-DB to blood vessels or other organ tissue. Massive 2.5-mmol doses injected into the carotid artery did suppress feeding.

Intravenous or intraperitoneal injection of 1.25 and 2.5 mmol 3,4-DB encapsulated in liposome vesicles significantly depressed feeding dose dependently. Probably 8% of the amount used was actually encapsulated (0.1 and 0.2 mmol), and 1% of this reached the brain (1 and 2 μmol). This amount reaching the brain was comparable to the effective intraventricular dose.

A physicochemical derivative of 3,4-DB is 2-B4O which has equal biological activity but increased lipophilicity. Interestingly, 2-B4O was initially synthesized for testing, but it was later isolated from blood serum. The effects of third ventricle injection of 2-B4O were similar in nature and in magnitude to those of 3,4-DB in both normal and 72-hr deprived rats. When administered intraperitoneally, 2-B4O significantly depressed feeding dose dependently for applications up to 0.4 mmol/kg. This amounts to about 0.13 mmol per animal, compared to the effective 0.1–0.2 mmol dose of 3,4-DB. Thus 2-B4O is biologically as active as 3,4-DB and is effective by central, peripheral, or oral application (*4*).

When the volume of rat cerebral spinal fluid (CSF) is about 300 μl, the concentrations of any of these sugar acids in CSF could be estimated at 4.2–8.3 mM after 1.2 to 2.5 μmol injection into the third ventricle if they were not metabolized. If CSF is produced at a rate of 0.5% of the total volume per minute, the concentration of sugar acids would be diluted to 22% of the initial concentration, 0.9–1.8 mM at about 5 hr after injection. The concentration of ketone bodies in CSF is about 50% of that in the blood (*3*) and increases from 0.12 to 1.6 mM after 96 hr food deprivation. This 1.6 mM value is similar to the 5 hr concentration estimated for the sugar acids. Because diffusion from the cerebral ventricle to the brain parenchyma is about 1% after 20 min, concentrations of 3,4-DB, 2-B4O, or 2,4,5-TP available to act in the LHA and VMH should be no more than 50–100 μM or 10–20 μM 5 hr after injection.

II. ELECTROPHYSIOLOGICAL EFFECTS OF SUGAR ACIDS ON GSNs AND GRNs

In anesthetized rats, electrophoretic application of 3,4-DB and 2-B4O suppressed and application of 2,4,5-TP enhanced GSN activ-

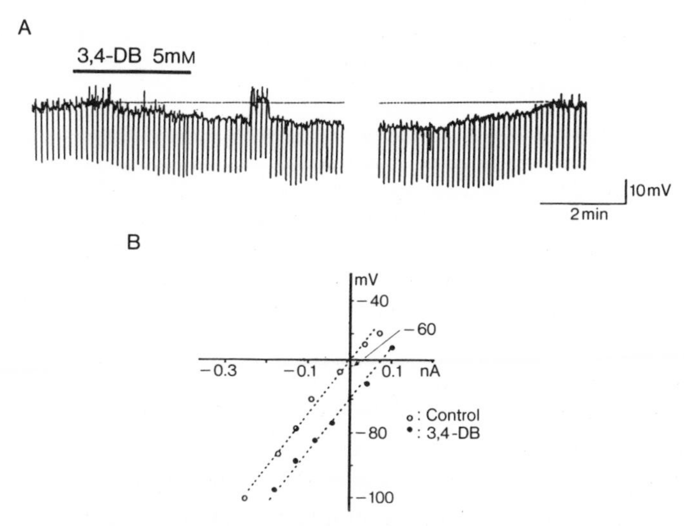

Fig. 2. Effect of 3,4-DB on rat LHA neuron. A: hyperpolarization by 9 mV during superfusion of 3,4-DB (5 mM) containing solution. Bars, superfusion time. Downward deflections, electrotonic potential amplitude by hyperpolarizing current pulse to measure input resistance. Restoration to the original membrane potential soon after end of 3,4-DB application revealed no remarkable change in input membrane resistance. Upward deflection, spontaneous action potentials (the full amplitude of which was not reproduced). B: current intensity-voltage (I-V) relationships during control (○) and 3,4-DB (5 mM) containing perfusion (●). These two parallel curves indicate no change in input membrane resistance before and during 3,4-DB application (*8*).

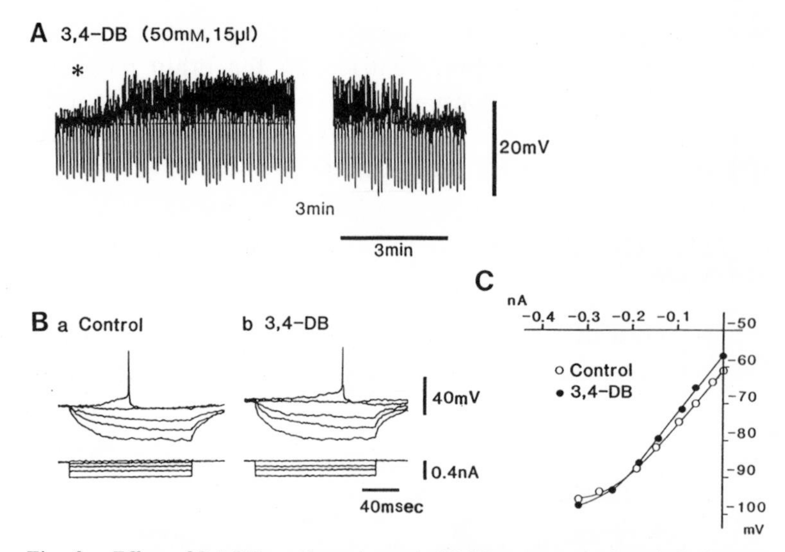

Fig. 3. Effect of 3,4-DB on the guinea pig VMH neuron. A: drop infusion (15 μl) of 50 mM 3,4-DB into an inlet reservoir depolarized membrane potential accompanied by an increase in firing frequency and input membrane resistance. B: actual response to various current pulses applied before and during 3,4-DB. Note increase in input membrane resistance by 3,4-DB (increased amplitudes by inward square current pulses). C: I-V plots of control (○) and 3,4-DB solution (●). Apparent reversal potential for the depolarization, −91 mV (*8*).

ity dose dependently. Effects of 3,4-DB, 2-B4O, or 2,4,5-TP on glucose-insensitive neurons (GINs) were negligible. Suppression of GSNs by 3,4-DB and by glucose was reversibly blocked by ouabain.

GRN activity was dose dependently inhibited by electrophoretic application of 2,4,5-TP and facilitated by 3,4-DB and 2-B4O (*3, 6, 7*). No non-GRNs were affected by any of these three compounds and no cortical neurons responded to electrophoretic application of 3,4-DB, 2-B4O or 2,4,5-TP.

The effects of 3,4-DB, 2-B4O, and 2,4,5-TP on membrane potentials and resistance were investigated in guinea pig and rat hypothalamic slice preparations (*7, 8*). Criteria for acceptable tests included maintenance of resting potential more negative than −50 mV, membrane input resistance above 80 MΩ, and membrane time

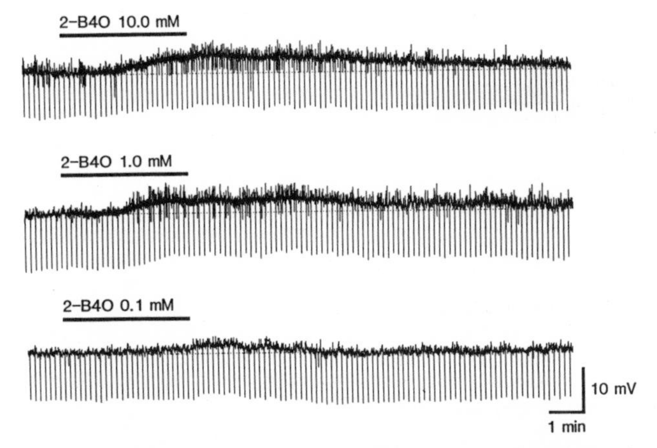

Fig. 4. Effect of 2-B4O on rat VMH neuron. Depolarizations in a dose dependent manner by perfusion of various concentrations of 2-B4O (0.1, 1.0, 10.0 mM) on same neuron. ---, resting potential (−55 mV). Downward deflections, electrotonic potential amplitude by constant current hyperpolarizing pulses passed through recording electrode to measure input membrane resistance. Note increase in the input membrane resistance by 2-B4O. Upward deflections and accompanying small downward deflections, spontaneous action potentials (full amplitude of which was not reproduced) and after-hyperpolarizations, respectively. Bars, super perfusion time of 2-B4O (*7*).

constant of at least 4 msec. GSNs in the LHA were hyperpolarized by 3,4-DB while membrane resistance remained constant (Fig. 2A). The reversal potential for 3,4-DB could not be obtained (Fig. 2B). Moreover, depression of the hyperpolarization by ouabain indicated that the effect of 3,4-DB, like that of glucose, was due to Na^+-K^+-pump activation through the action of ATP. In the VMH, GRNs were depolarized by 3,4-DB and 2-B4O while membrane resistance increased (Fig. 3A, B; Fig. 4). The reversal potential for 3,4-DB and 2-B4O depolarizations was about −90 mV, close to the K^+ equilibrium potential (Fig. 3C, Fig. 5). Since this result was the same as that produced by glucose, depolarization by glucose and that by 3,4-DB and 2-B4O are both caused by K^+ permeability decrease (*9*). These results also suggest that 3,4-DB and 2-B4O are metabolized in

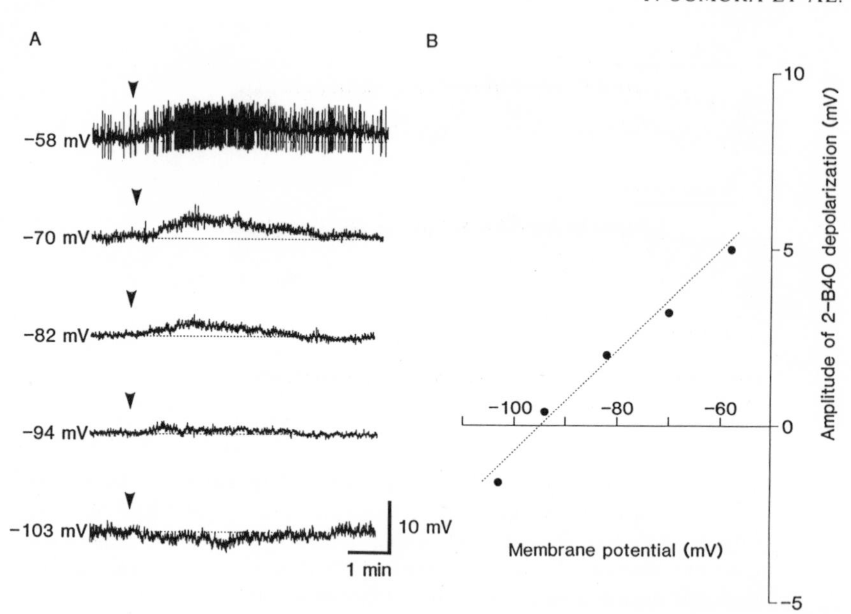

Fig. 5. Measurement of reversal potential for depolarization by 2-B4O on rat VMH neuron. A: responses to 2-B4O, recorded at different membrane potential. Depolarization, reversed to hyperpolarization by passing current between −94 and −103 mV. ▾ application of 2-B4O (50 mM) as a drop. B: plots of values obtained in A. Reversal potential for 2-B4O depolarization, −95 mV (7).

the brain, the same as ketone bodies, if there is a shortage of glucose.

Facilitation of GSN activity by 2,4,5-TP was caused by membrane depolarization with membrane resistance decrease (Fig. 6A). The reversal potential for depolarization was about +40 mV, close to the Na^+ equilibrium potential (Fig. 6B). Inhibition of GRN activity by 2,4,5-TP was due to hyperpolarization with membrane resistance decreases (Fig. 7A, B). The reversal potential for hyperpolarization was about −90 mV, showing that 2,4,5-TP increased membrane K^+ permeability (Fig. 7C).

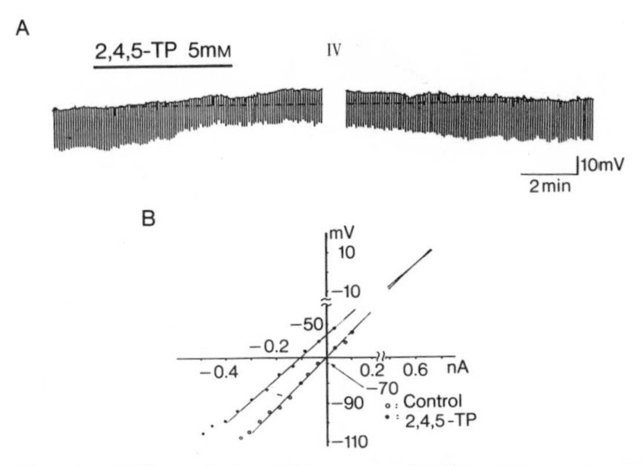

Fig. 6. Effect of 2,4,5-TP on rat LHA neuron. A: superfusion with 5 mM 2,4,5-TP produced 10 mV depolarization associated with a decrease in input membrane resistance. B: relation of I-V plots of control (○) and 2,4,5-TP application (●). Estimated reversal potential, +10 mV (*7*).

III. PERIPHERAL EFFECT OF THE SUGAR ACIDS

Levels of plasma glucose and insulin were changed by injections of 2.5 μmol 3,4-DB, 2-B4O, and 2,4,5-TP into the rat third ventricle (*4*). Blood glucose was increased about 20% by 3,4-DB, first transiently and then continuously for 8 hr. Insulin concentration was only slightly affected by 3,4-DB. Glucose was depressed 20% by 2,4,5-TP, but recovered later. Insulin level increased to 2.6 times control. The increase in insulin level induced by 2,4,5-TP agrees with increased vagal efferent activity and decreased splanchnic efferent activity to the pancreas that appear after 2,4,5-TP induced increased LHA activity and decreased VMH activity (*11, 12*).

Blood glucose was increased dose-dependently and to 1.3 times control for about 4 hr by intraperitoneal injection of 30 μmol/kg 2-B4O (Fig. 8). During that time, vagal efferent activity to the pancreas and liver decreased and splanchnic efferent activity to the pancreas, liver, adrenal gland, kidney, and brown adipose tissue increased for 3 hr by 25 nmol, 2-B4O intravenous injection. The plasma corticosterone also increased in a dose dependent manner, 0.28 μg/ml to 0.45 μg/ml by an intravenous injection of 30 μmol/

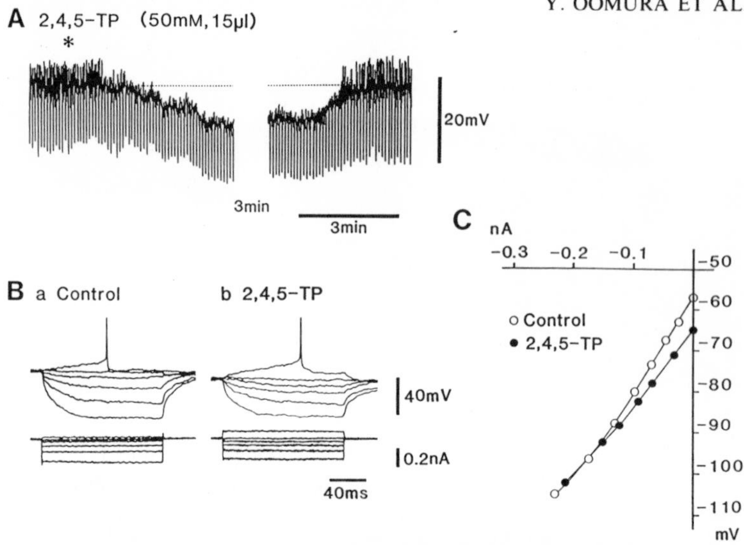

Fig. 7. Effect of 2,4,5-TP on the guinea pig VMH neuron. A : drop infusion (15 μl) of 50mM 2,4,5-TP hyperpolarized the membrane potential and decreased the input membrane resistance. B : actual responses to various pulses before and during 2,4,5-TP. Note decreases in input membrane resistance by 2,4,5-TP (decreased amplitudes by inward current pulses). C: I-V plots of control (○) and 2,4,5-TP (●) solution. Apparent reversal potential for hyperpolarization, −96 mV (*7*).

kg 2-B4O. This increase was attenuated not by the cut of the splanchnic adrenal nerve but by anti CRF antibody application (Fig. 9).

Changes induced in plasma levels of glucose and insulin by 3,4-DB, 2-B4O, and 2,4,5-TP were consistent with the effect that each substance has on feeding behavior. Gastric acid secretion induced by 2-deoxy-D-glucose was suppressed by application of 3,4-DB or 2-B4O in the LHA, and secretion was elicited by 2,4,5-TP applied the same way (*13*).

SUMMARY

These sugar acids appear to modulate feeding behavior by modifying LHA and VMH neuronal activity. Substances such as

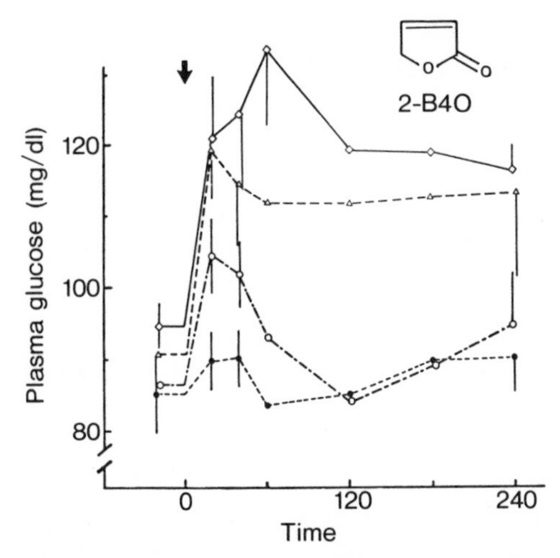

Fig. 8. Increase in plasma glucose concentration by 2-B4O intraperitoneal injection. ● saline ($n=5$); ○ 3 μmol/kg ($n=5$); △ 30 μmol/kg ($n=6$); ◇ 300 μmol/kg ($n=5$). Mean±SE.

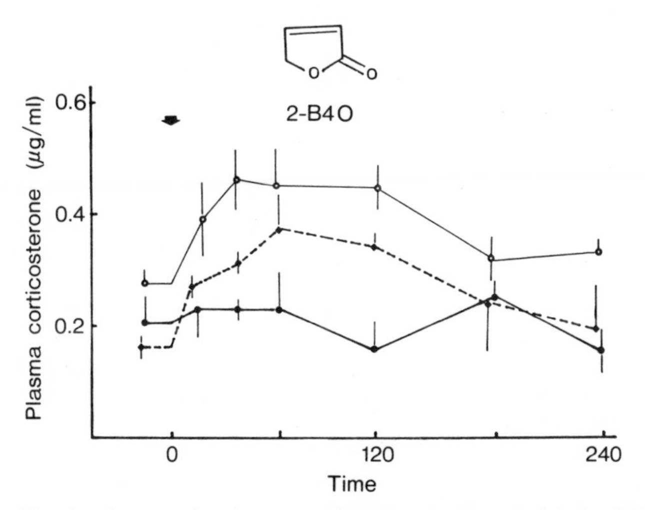

Fig. 9. Increase in plasma corticosterone concentration by 2-B4O intraperitoneal injection (30 μmol/kg). Control (○). Cut of splanchnic adrenal nerve (♦) had no effect. Antibody of CRF intraperitoneal injection (●) attenuated the increase in plasma corticosterone.

calcitonin and glucagon mimic glucose in the rat LHA. Hypothalamic GRNs and GSNs, which receive information from many humoral sources, are important in the regulation of feeding. These sugar acids modify plasma glucose, insulin, corticosterone levels, and feeding behavior. It is suggested that 2,4,5-TP is a hunger-inducing substance and 3,4-DB and 2-B4O induce the sensation of satiety through their effects on the activity of GSNs and GRNs.

Acknowledgment

We thank Prof. A. Simpson for help with the manuscript.

REFERENCES

1. Oomura, Y., Ono, T., Ooyama, H., and Wayner, M.J. (1969). Glucose and osmosensitive neurones of the rat hypothalamus. *Nature* **222**, 282–284.
2. Oomura, Y. (1987). Role of chemical substances in the control of food intake. *In* "Advances in Physiological Research," McLennan, H., Ledsome, J.R., McIntosh, C.H.S., and Jones, D.R., eds., pp. 331–375. Plenum Press, New York.
3. Shimizu, N., Oomura, Y., and Sakata, T. (1984). Modulation of feeding by endogenous sugar acids acting as hunger or satiety factors. *Am. J. Physiol.* **246**, R532–R550.
4. Plata-Salaman, G.R., Oomura, Y., and Shimizu, N. (1986). Endogenous sugar acid derivative acting as a feeding suppressant. *Physiol. Behav.* **38**, 359–373.
5. Oomura, Y. (1987). Regulation of feeding by neural responses to endogenous factors. *News Physiol. Sci.* **2**, 197–203.
6. Puthuraya, K.P., Oomura, Y., and Shimizu, N. (1985). Effects of endogenous sugar acids on the ventromedial hypothalamic nucleus of the rat. *Brain Res.* **332**, 165–168.
7. Fukuda, A., Oomura, Y., Minami, T., and Ito, C. (1988). A novel endogenous sugar acid depolarizes ventromedial hypothalamic neurons *in vitro. Am. J. Physiol.* **255**, R134–R140.
8. Minami, T., Oomura, Y., Nabekura, J., and Fukuda, A. (1988). Direct effects of 3,4-dihydrobutanoic acid γ-lactone on lateral and ventromedial hypothalamic neurons. *Brain Res.*, in press.
9. Minami, T., Oomura, Y., and Sugimori, M. (1986). Electrophysiological properties and glucose responsiveness of guinea-pig ventromedial hypothalamic neurones *in vitro. J. Physiol.* **380**, 127–143.
10. Oomura, Y. (1986). Feeding regulation by endogenous sugar acids through hypothalamic chemosensitive neurons. *Brain Res. Bull.* **17**, 551–562.
11. Oomura, Y. and Kita, H. (1981). Insulin acting as a modulator of feeding through

the hypothalamus. *Diabetologia* **20**, 290–298.
12. Yoshimatsu, H., Niijima, A., Oomura, Y., Yamabe, K., and Katafuchi, T. (1984). Effects of hypothalamic lesion on pancreatic autonomic nerve activity in the rat. *Brain Res.* **303**, 147–152.
13. Shiraishi, T., Kawashima, M., and Oomura, Y. (1985). Endogenous sugar acid control of hypothalamic neuron activity and gastric acid secretion in rats. *Brain Res. Bull.* **14**, 431–438.

Diet and Obesity, Bray, G.A. et al., eds., pp. 17-35.
Japan Sci. Soc. Press, Tokyo/S. Karger, Basel (1988)

Controls of Food Intake and Energy Expenditure

GEORGE A. BRAY

Department of Medicine, University of Southern California, School of Medicine, Los Angeles, CA 90033, U.S.A.

Obesity is an outward reflection of increased nutrients stored as fat. For young men a body fat above 25% is obese; for young women a comparable figure is 30%. Why does this positive nutrient balance occur? It implies a disturbance in a system which is normally regulated. A regulated system has several features. First, there is a controller located in the brain. Second, there is a controlled system consisting of food intake, its storage, and metabolism. Third, there are feedback elements which tell the controller about the controlled system, and finally there are the efferent control mechanisms.

The regulatory system for body weight is often considered to be controlling energy balance *per se* (*1, 2*). However, a more detailed analysis suggests that each individual macronutrient is regulated separately. Many elements of the regulatory systems for energy or nutrient balance appear to operate across species. Although species variations obviously exist, the basic neurochemical and physiological mechanisms appear to apply to most mammalian species (*3*).

In analyzing a controlled or regulated system we can begin from either the controlled system, the controller, the feedback signals or the efferent control elements. This analysis will begin with the controlled system and end with the efferent controls.

I. CONTROLLED NUTRIENT SYSTEM

The controlled or regulated system for nutrient balance is concerned with maintenance of appropriate nutrient stores of each macronutrient. In addition to water, which is the major constituent of all living cells and is closely regulated, the controlled system for macronutrients includes the intake, storage, and disposal of protein, carbohydrate, and fat.

In a normal human being total body fat stores are approximately 140,000 kcal (588MJ) (*2, 3*). This is some six times the quantity of energy that is stored as protein (24,000 kcal or 100.8MJ). By comparison, the quantity of carbohydrate available as glycogen stores from liver, kidney, muscle, and other tissues plus the glucose that circulates in the blood is minute, equivalent to only 800 kcal (3. 36MJ). Figure 1 shows the typical intake of 2,000 kcal (8.4MJ) as protein, carbohydrate and fat with a 20/40/40% distribution. The adjacent bars represent the percentage of the daily intake related to

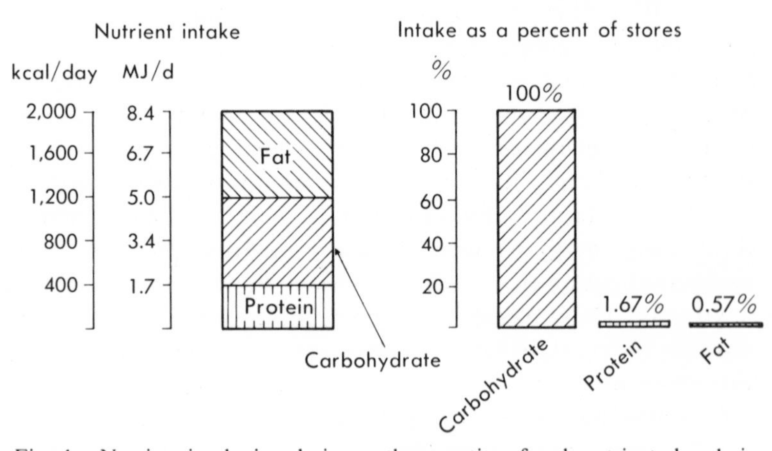

Fig. 1. Nutrient intake in relation to the quantity of each nutrient already in body stores.

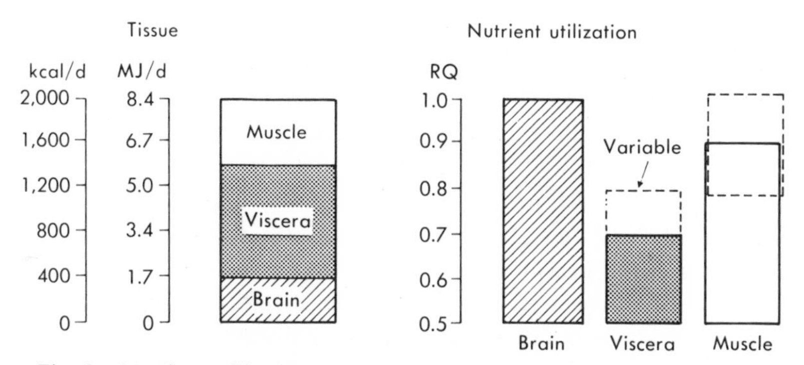

Fig. 2. Nutrient utilization at rest. The participation of energy between the various tissues is shown at the left, and the relative quantities of carbohydrate and fat, as the respiratory quotient, are shown on the right. An RQ of 1 is a tissue which is oxidizing 100% carbohydrate, and an RQ of 0.7 is a tissue which is oxidizing 100% fat. Viscera and muscle are depicted as showing some adaptability in relation to diet.

the preexisting energy stores for each component. It is clear that carbohydrate intake at 800 kcal/day (200 g) is equal to 100% of the body stores of carbohydate. On the other hand, protein intake is only a little over 1% of total stores, and fat intake is less than 1%. It is not surprising, therefore, that in studies of nutrient balance in experimental animals Flatt (*4*) has noted that changes in carbohydrate balance from day to day influence changes in carbohydrate intake on the subsequent day. For fat balance, on the other hand, the day-to-day relationship has a very shallow slope indicating that daily fat balance has much less effect on subsequent fat (food) intake.

A second feature of the regulatory system is shown in Fig. 2. Energy utilization by various tissues at rest is partitioned into the fraction utilized by muscle, viscera, and brain. Muscle and skin account for approximately 18% of energy expenditure at rest, but this can increase to more than 50% during locomotion (physical activity) (*5*). Brain and visceral metabolism, on the other hand, represent a much larger fraction of basal or resting component of energy expenditure and are much less variable in absolute amounts. The relative contribution of each of these tissues to oxidation of carbohydrate and fat, expressed as the respiratory quotient (RQ), is shown in the right-hand three bars. Brain oxidizes primarily glucose and at 20% of total daily energy expenditure represents an organ which burns 100% carbohydrate and thus has an RQ of 1. Visceral tissues, on the other hand, are predominantly consumers of fatty acids or ketones and utilize only small quantities of carbohydrate which may vary to a small extent with diet or exercise (as shown schematically by the dashed areas in Fig. 2). Muscle utilizes variable quantities of carbohydrate and fat, depending on its state of training and the intensity and duration of exercise. During short bouts of intense exercise carbohydrate provides the major fuel and is mobilized in large part from glycogen stores within muscle. During more prolonged exercise of an aerobic nature the percentage of fatty acids oxidized by muscle increases and the RQ falls. One major difference between the physically trained muscle and the untrained muscle is its ability to oxidize fatty acids during exercise and at rest. These basic facts about the nutrient control system can be summarized in the following equation.

$$\text{Nutrient balance} = \sum[(\Delta\text{carbohydrate balance}) + (\Delta\text{fat balance}) + \Delta\text{protein balance})]$$

Several hypotheses are suggested by this equation:

1. That the balance of each major nutrient may be regulated separately.

2. That the time required to achieve balance varies for each nutrient as a function of the amount ingested each day in relation to the total body stores. Thus becoming obese by eating a high carbohydrate diet would appear to be more difficult than with a fat diet (*6*) because the body storage systems for carbohydrate are limited. Although excess carbohydrate can be converted to fatty acids, this is an energetically expensive transformation. Body fat stores, on the other hand, are many times larger than fat intake implying a much greater storage capacity for fat and a much longer time constant to achieve balance.

3. That achievement of nutrient balance requires that the net

oxidation of each nutrient equals the average composition of the nutrients in the diet.

4. That ingestion of a high fat diet requires greater fat oxidation than a low fat diet.

5. That since physical training can increase the oxidation of fatty acids by muscle, regular aerobic exercise might reduce the tendency to become obese on a higher fat diet.

6. Finally, that the regulation of nutrient stores is subject to positive and negative feedback elements for each component which operates through the central controller.

Nutrient intake plays a variable role in the development of experimental forms of obesity (*7, 8*) and thus probably in human obesity as well. This is presented graphically in Fig. 3. This is a three dimensional representation to show, along the X-axis, the dependence of obesity on dietary composition and whether hyperphagia is present or not and whether that hyperphagia is essential for the development of obesity. It can be seen that the animals with lesions in the paraventricular nucleus (PVN) (*9, 10*) are hyper-

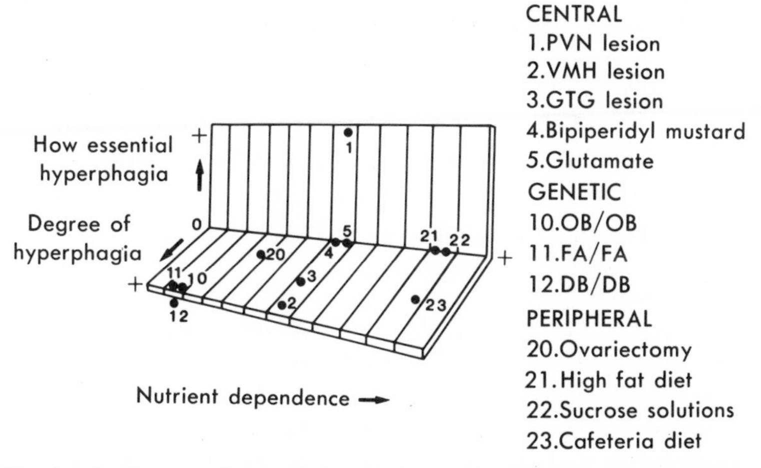

Fig. 3. A diagram of the relative nutrient dependence of various animal models of obesity. Also shown is the dependence and presence of these models of hyperphagia for the appearance of obesity.

phagic and that this appears to be essential for the development of this syndrome (*11*). However, development of obesity in animals with PVN-lesions appears to be relatively independent of the nutrient composition of the diet, *i.e.*, they will become fat on high or low carbohydrate diets. The other forms of hypothalamic obesity produced by lesions in the ventromedial hypothalamus or by injecting gold thioglucose are no more nutrient dependent than PVN-lesioned animals (*7*). They also have hyperphagia but this hyperphagia is not essential for the development of these syndromes (*12, 13*). Two other syndromes with hypothalamic injury, that due to the injection of bipiperidyl mustard or monosodium glutamate (No. 4 and 5) are not hyperphagic and will become obese on any diet. The genetic obesities (No. 10–12) are all hyperphagic but this hyperphagia is not essential for the development of obesity in these animals (*7, 14, 15*). Moreover, animals with genetic obesity will become fat on high or low carbohydrate diets. Of syndromes due to peripheral manipulations, ovariectomy shows modest hyperphagia which is not essential for development of this syndrome, but these animals are more susceptible to a high fat diet (*8*). High fat diets (*16*), access to sucrose solutions (*17*), and cafeteria diets (*18*) have a high nutrient dependence for the development of obesity. Of these types of dietary obesity, cafeteria-fed rats are the most hyperphagic while the other two show only limited degrees of hyperphagia. This review of animal models shows that nutrient dependence and hyperphagia are separable dimensions in the equation for obesity.

II. THE BRAIN AS CONTROLLER

1. Anatomy

Several anatomic regions of the brain appear to play an important role in the control of nutrient balance (*19*). Destruction of the ventromedial hypothalamus is associated with increased fat stores in most homeothermic species which have been studied (*7*). On the other hand, destruction of regions in the lateral hypothalamus is associated with a reduction in body fat. More recently the PVN has been shown to be a particularly important region for stimulation of food intake following topical injection of both norepinephrine (*20*) and such neuropeptides as dynorphin (*20*), and neuropeptide Y (*20*). The primacy of the ventromedial nucleus in the regulation of body fat stores is suggested by the fact that the chronic infusion of norepinephrine into the ventromedial hypothalamus produces obesity, whereas comparable infusion into the PVN does not have this effect (*21*).

2. Neurotransmitters

Norepinephrine, serotonin, and several peptides may be involved in the transmission of information which regulates food intake and nutrient stores. As noted above, hypothalamic norepinephrine infusions can increase fat stores (*21*). Serotonin also plays an important role in the regulation of food intake and nutrient stores (*22*). Tryptophan and 5-hydroxytryptophan, two precursors of serotonin, both decrease food intake (*23*). Drugs which block the effect of serotonin can increase body weight and those which stimulate the release of serotonin or inhibit its re-uptake from nerve endings will result in a reduction in body weight. Thus, norepinephrine and serotonin appear to play important roles in the regulation of food intake through structures located in the medial and lateral hypothalamus.

Several peptides also modulate food intake and may influence nutrient storage (*20, 24, 25*). Neuropeptide Y, beta-endorphin, dynorphin, and galanin can all stimulate food intake when applied to the ventromedial or PVN (*20, 26*). On the other hand, a variety of peptides including bombesin, cholecystokinin, neurotensin, somatostatin, and corticotropin-releasing factor (CRF) can inhibit feeding when injected topically in the region of the ventromedial nucleus or when infused into the third ventricular system (*20, 24, 25*). In addition to these neuropeptides there is also evidence to suggest that raising the concentration of insulin within the cerebral spinal fluid can decrease food intake in several species, but the physiological importance of this remains unclear (*27, 28*).

III. FEEDBACK SIGNALS

The central neurotransmitters involved in regulating nutrient balance are activated by afferent signals transmitted through the blood or over the autonomic or sensory nervous system. As noted above, carbohydrate balance appears to be regulated on a day-to-day basis in mice (*4*). Since carbohydrate stores are concentrated as glycogen in muscle and liver, one reasonable mechanism for modulation of carbohydrate balance would be through hepatic glycogen stores. Glucoreceptors in the liver can transmit information to the brain through vagal afferent nerves (*29*). Vagal afferent nerve fibers have been traced from the liver to the nucleus of the tractus solaritarius (NTS) and from there through the parabrachial nucleus to the lateral hypothalamus and then to the PVN (*30*). Cholecystokinin, which inhibits food intake in man and animals (*24*), may be involved in this afferent vagal system, since it is ineffective in lowering food intake after vagotomy or with lesions in the nucleus of the tractus solitarius or PVN. Glucagon also requires an intact afferent vagal system to induce satiety. These data suggest that the afferent vagal circuitry may be one way in which changes in glucose balance might modulate food intake through the PVN. A second possible mechanism is through direct effects of glucose on the central nervous system (*30*). Hauger *et al.* (*32*) have demonstrated that glucose regulates the binding of amphetamine to the sodium pump (Na^+-K^+ ATPase) in the hypothalamus, and that this effect is modulated by nutrient intake, specifically glucose. Thus at least two mechanisms may be involved in the regulation of glucose balance.

The potential role for serotonin in the regulation of protein intake and/or carbohydrate balance is suggested by the relationship between tryptophan and food intake (*23*). Tryptophan, 5-hydroxytryptophan, and drugs like fenfluramine (*33*), which increase serotonin concentrations at neuroeffector junctions are known to alter the preference for carbohydrates and modify the preference for protein while those which influence the noradrenergic system, specifically amphetamines, alter the preference for protein (*33*).

Fat balance provides a more complicated problem. Increasing the percentage of fat in the diet will increase body fat stores in animal species (*16*). However, within each species there are some members which are considerably more resistant to developing obesity when eating a high fat diet than others.

In our studies on sensitive and resistant variants of rats fed a high fat diet, we have observed that the resistant rats have a number of important differences in their response to a high fat diet when compared to the sensitive rats. Changes of food intake in response to insulin and anorectic drugs were significantly different (*34*). Blood levels of ketones were increased in the resistant rats and may be a reflection of the changes in insulin concentrations. Ketones are the metabolic product of fatty acid metabolism by the liver, and are secreted for transport to other tissues where they provide an important metabolic fuel. Ketones may also provide a signal to the liver or brain about the state of fatty acid oxidization. We have observed that the transport of 3-hydroxybutyrate across the blood brain barrier is significantly higher in the rats which are resistant to dietary obesity than in the animals which are sensitive to high fat diet (*35*). When animals are fed a high fat diet, there is an increase in blood brain barrier transport mechanisms but the resistant animals still transport significantly more than the sensitive ones (*35*). In other studies from our laboratory we have observed that the infusion of ketones into the ventricular system of the brain enhances sympathetic activity as reflected by the increased thermogenic properties of brown adipose tissue (BAT) (*36*) and by the increased sympathetic firing rate of nerves to BAT when ketones are microinjected into the ventromedial hypothalamus (VMH) (*37*). This is in harmony with the observations of Davis *et al.* (*38*) and suggests that the VMH plays a pivotal role in producing resistance to obesity in rats eating a high fat diet.

The importance of the ventromedial hypothalamus in the resistant rat is underlined by the fact that VMH lesions convert the resistant rat into one that is sensitive to a high fat diet (*39*). The resistant rats also show an altered pattern of response to drugs which attenuate food intake (*34*) but not to castration or sucrose-induced obesity (*40*).

Differences in efferent controls also exist between resistant and sensitive rats. The resistant animal has a higher activity of its sympathetic nervous system than the animal which is sensitive to a high fat diet (*41*). Since the concentration of ketones available to the brain tissue is a function of the rate of transport across the blood brain barrier the resistant strain should, and does have, increased activity of the sympathetic nervous system. It is of interest that the response to ketones infused into the cerebroventricular system does not appear to vary with the diet. Thus a higher blood brain barrier transport of ketones following exposure to a high fat diet would lead to greater quantities of ketones in the brain and subsequently to greater activation of the sympathetic nervous system by this mechanism.

IV. EFFERENT CONTROLS

The final section of the nutrient control model for obesity is the efferent controls. One of these efferent controls is the complex sequence of motor activities which leads to the initiation of food seeking, and the killing and/or ingestion of the food. These areas seem to be integrated in the lateral hypothalamus, since electrical stimulation of this area will lead to ingestive behavior.

1. Autonomic Nervous System

Another group of efferent controls deals with internal regulators which are related to changes in nutrient intake and stores. In animals where obesity follows hypothalamic lesions, there is evidence for increased activity of the vagal system (*7, 42–44*). This provides one of the explanations for the increase in insulin which characterizes this syndrome. However, reduction in sympathetic activity may be more characteristic of the obese state and may enhance insulin secretion (*45–47*). The activity of the sympathetic nervous system is normally increased in response to sucrose (*48*) or glucose (*49*). In the experimental animal, there appears to be an inverse relationship between the activity of the sympathetic nervous system and food intake (*50*). During spontaneous eating, the correlation between basal activity of the sympathetic nervous system and food intake is $r = -0.91$. In addition, most of the experimental maneuvers we have tested which increase food intake result in a decrease in the activity of the sympathetic nervous system. Two apparent exceptions to this relationship are observed in fasted animals (*48*), and in animals eating a cafeteria or supermarket diet (*51*). In fasted rats, the activity of the sympathetic system declines (*48, 52*). However, this reduction in the sympathetic activity may be consistent with the negative correlation between food intake and sympathetic activity, if one views the level of food intake of the fasted animal by asking how much the animal would have eaten if food were available. With our model of a negative correlation between food intake and resting sympathetic activity, the low sympathetic activity observed with fasting would predict an increased level of food intake when food first becomes available. Van Itallie and Kissileff (*53*) have observed precisely this relationship with a higher initial level of food intake as the degree of fasting is prolonged.

The increased food intake of the cafeteria fed rat (*51*), or the

TABLE I
Factors Affecting Sympathetic Activity

Physiologic variable	Sympathetic activity		
	Low	Normal	High
Hypothalamic lesion	VMH	PVN	LH
Food intake—quality	High fat	Mixed diet	High carbohydrate
Food intake—quantity	Fasting	Average	Overeating
Genetic obesity	FA/FA	+/?	
	OB/OB	+/?	
	DB/DB	+/?	
Corticosteroid level	High		Low (ADX)
Insulin level	Low		High
Thyroid hormone level	High		Low
Temperature	Hot	Neutral	Cold
Lactation	Lactating		

LH, lateral hypothalamus; FA, fatty; OB, obese; DB, diabetic; ADX, adrenalectomy.

animal drinking sucrose solutions (*54*) may represent positive feedback signals which may override the normal reciprocal relationship between food intake and the sympathetic nervous system.

The effects of various maneuvers on the sympathetic nervous system are summarized in Table I. It is clear that this system plays an important role in the regulation of a variety of basic bodily functions as well as its adaptive response to a variety of signals. The effects of adrenalectomy discussed below play an important role in the activity of the sympathetic nervous system and its participation in the regulation of nutrient control.

2. Adrenal Steroids

The development or progression of experimental obesity is reversed or attenuated by adrenalectomy (*55–57*). This striking observation requires special consideration. The fact that almost all defects in the genetically obese animal are reversed by adrenalectomy (*58–62*) suggested that glucocorticoids might play a key role in the development of this syndrome. Adrenalectomy produces two effects on nutrient balance (*63*). First, nutrient intake returns nearly, if not completely, to normal levels after adrenalectomy in genetically obese animals, in those with castration-induced obesity (*57*) and in those with hypothalamic obesity (*46*). Feeding patterns also revert to normal (*60*). Leibowitz (*20*) has described one way in which feeding may be influenced by adrenalectomy. She has shown that adrenalectomy almost completely abolishes the stimulation of food intake when norepinephrine is injected into the PVN (*20*). Treatment with corticosterone rapidly reverses this effect. This loss of sensitivity after adrenalectomy could explain the return of food intake to normal after adrenalectomy.

Energy expenditure is also increased after adrenalectomy (*61, 62, 64*). We (*64*) and others (*61, 65*) have shown increased activity of the sympathetic nervous system as measured by increased norepinephrine turnover in nerve endings in brown adipose tissue (*64*) as well as increased binding of guanosine 5′-diphosphate to mitochondria from this tissue as an index of thermogenic activity (*62*) in response to adrenalectomy. The effects of corticosteroids on ther-

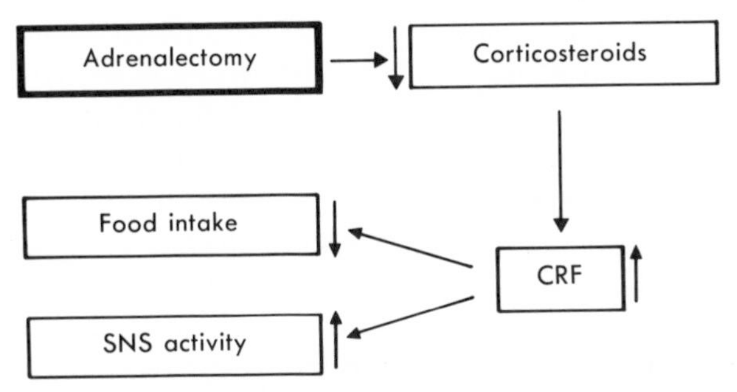

Fig. 4. A model of the effects of adrenalectomy in the control of sympathetic nervous activity and food intake. The central actor in this system is the CRF which can modulate the reciprocal changes in food intake and sympathetic activity.

mogenic activity can be observed in normal (*63*) as well as obese animals (*62*).

Since efferent systems for food intake and sympathetic activity are affected by adrenalectomy, the effect of removing glucocorticoids would appear to act at a site different from the ones involved in genetic obesity, dietary obesity, or hypothalamic obesity. After adrenalectomy, the negative feedback signal produced by corticosterone is absent and CRF will be released into the hypothalamic portal circulation to stimulate increased adrenocorticotropic hormone (ACTH) output from the pituitary. This increased CRF may also serve as the principle stimulus for the reduction of food intake and for the increased sympathetic activity following adrenalectomy. Injections of CRF into the ventricle of the rat decrease food intake (*66, 67*) and increase circulating levels of epinephrine and norepinephrine (*68*). Since adrenalectomy attenuates obesity in genetically obese animals, this would suggest that the mechanism by which CRF works is different for both food intake and sympathetic activity from those mechanisms associated with any of the other neurotransmitter systems involved in the syndromes of hypothalamic, genetic or dietary obesity. This hypothesis is presented schematically in Fig. 4.

This review has looked at nutrient intake as a regulated system.

The principle feedback elements involve vagal afferent fibers from the liver, stomach, and pancreas. Nutrients from food including ketones produced by oxidation of fatty acids in the liver as well as circulating hormones released by the process of ingestion, digestion, and storage of nutrients may also provide negative feedback signals to the brain. In addition, positive feedback elements are associated with the smell and taste of food. Social occasions and other events which lead to overriding the normal satiety mechanisms can lead to enhanced food intake. Within the controller are the receptor systems for the integration of messages that under normal circumstances control the feeding system. The lateral and ventromedial hypothalamus act reciprocally to control the parasympathetic and sympathetic system. Following adrenalectomy, CRF increases and may override the defects of genetic and hypothalamic obesity. Such a model provides new insights into potential therapeutic approaches to obesity by developing strategies to modulate each nutrient. The concept that nutrient balance is regulated by controlling the balance of individual nutrients provides important advice today on the type of diet and importance of exercise in the regulation of obesity:

1. Eat a high-carbohydrate, low-fat diet.
2. Exercise to maintain muscles at moderate degrees of training.

SUMMARY

The regulation of body energy stores is considered to be a controlled system. Such a system has a controller located in the brain, afferent signals from peripheral sites, efferent signals which arise from the brain after integrating information from the periphery as well as internal signals, and a controlled system consisting of the storage, metabolism, and utilization of nutrient energy. The thesis of this paper is that each major macronutrient, protein, carbohydrate and fat, is regulated separately. Two implications of this analysis of the food control system is that people should eat a high-carbohydrate low-fat diet, and that they should exercise to maintain muscles at moderate degrees of training.

Acknowledgement

This work was supported in part by Grant RO1-DK32018 from the National Institute of Health, Regulation of Energy Balance.

REFERENCES

1. Woo, R., Daniels-Kush, R., and Horton, E.S. (1984). Regulation of energy balance. *Annu. Rev. Nutr.* **5**, 411-433.
2. Garrow, J.S. (1978). "Energy Balance and Obesity in Man," 2nd Edition. Elsevier/North-Holland Biomedical Press, Amsterdam.
3. Bray, G.A. (1987). Obesity—A disease of nutrient or energy balance? *Nutr. Rev.* **45**, 33-43.
4. Flatt, P.R. (1987). Dietary fat, carbohydrate balance, and weight maintenance: effects of exercise. *Am. J. Clin. Nutr.* **45**, 296-306.
5. Carlson, L.D. and Hsieh, A.C.L. (1970). "The Control of Energy Exchange." The MacMillan Co., New York.
6. Donato, K. and Hegsted, D.M. (1985). Efficiency of utilization of various sources of energy for growth. *Proc. Natl. Acad. Sci. U.S.A.* **82**, 4866-4870.
7. Bray, G.A. and York, D.A. (1979). Hypothalamic and genetic obesity in experimental animals: an autonomic and endocrine hypothesis. *Physiol. Rev.* **59**, 719-809.
8. Sclafani, A. (1984). Animal models of obesity: classification and characterization. *Int. J. Obesity* **8**, 491-508.
9. Tokunaga, K., Fukushima, M., Kemnitz, J.W., and Bray, G.A. (1986). Comparison of ventromedial and paraventricular lesions in rats that become obese. *Am. J. Physiol.* **251**, R1221-R1227.
10. Leibowitz, S.F., Hammer, N.J., and Chang, K. (1981). Hypothalamic paraventricular nucleus lesions produce overeating and obesity in the rat. *Physiol. Behav.* **27**, 1031-1040.
11. Weingarten, J.P., Chang, P., and McDonald, T.J. (1985). Comparison of the metabolic and behavioral disturbances following paraventricular and ventromedial hypothalamic lesions. *Brain Res. Bull.* **14**, 551-559.
12. Han, P.W. and Frohman, L.A. (1970). Hyperinsulinemia in tube-fed hypophysectomized rats bearing hypothalamic lesions. *Am. J. Physiol.* **219**, 1632-1636.
13. Frohman, L.A., Bernardis, L.L., Schnatz, J.D., and Burek, L. (1969). Plasma insulin and triglyceride levels after hypothalamic lesions in weanling rats. *Am. J. Physiol.* **216**, 1496-1501.
14. Coleman, D.L. (1982). Thermogenesis in diabetes-obesity syndromes in mutant mice. *Diabetologia* **22**, 205-211.
15. Cox, J.E. and Powley, T.L. (1977). Development of obesity in diabetic mice pair-fed with lean siblings. *J. Comp. Physiol. Psychol.* **91**, 347-358.

16. Schemmel, R., Mickelson, O., and Gill, J.L. (1970). Dietary obesity in rats. Body weight and body fat accretion in seen strains of rats. *J. Nutr.* **100**, 1041–1048.
17. Kanarek, R.B. and Hirsch, E. (1977). Dietary-induced overeating in experimental animals. *Fed. Proc.* **36**, 154–158.
18. Rothwell, N.J. and Stock, M.J. (1979). A role for brown adipose tissue in diet-induced thermogenesis. *Nature* **281**, 31–35.
19. Luiten, P.G.M., ter Horst, G.J., and Steffens, A.B. (1987). The hypothalamus, intrinsic connections and outflow pathways to the endocrine system in relation to the control of feeding and metabolism. *Prog. Neurobiol.* **28**, 1–54.
20. Leibowitz, S.F. (1986). Brain monoamines and peptides: roles in the control of eating behavior. *Fed. Proc.* **45**, 1396–1403.
21. Shimazu, T., Noama, M., and Saito, M. (1986). Chronic infusion of norepinephrine into the ventromedial hypothalamus induced obesity in rats. *Brain Res.* **369**, 215–223.
22. Blundell, J.E. (1984). Serotonin and appetite. *Neuropharmacology* **23**, 1537–1552.
23. Wurtman, R.J. and Wurtman, J.J, (1984). Nutrients, neurotransmitter synthesis, and the control of food intake. *In* "Eating and its Disorders," Stunkard, A.J. and Stellard, E., eds., pp. 77–96. Raven Press, New York.
24. Baile, C.A., McLaughlin, C.L., and Della-Fera, M.A. (1986). Role of cholecystokinin and opioid peptides in the control of food intake. *Physiol. Rev.* **66**, 172–234.
25. Morley, J.E. and Levine, A.S. (1985). The pharmacology of eating behavior. *Annu.Rev. Pharmacol. Toxicol.* **25**, 127–146.
26. Morley, J.E. and Levine, A.S. (1981). Dynorphin (1-3) induces spontaneous feeding in rats. *Life Sci.* **29**, 1901–1903.
27. Woods, S.C., Lotter, E.C., McKay, L.D., and Porte, D., Jr. (1979). Chronic intracerebroventricular infusion of insulin reduces food intake and body weight of baboons. *Nature* **282**, 503–505.
28. Brief, D.J. and Davis, J.D. (1984). Reduction of food intake and body weight by chronic intraventricular insulin infusion. *Brain Res. Bull.* **12**, 571–575.
29. Niijima, A. (1984). The effect of D-glucose on the firing rate of glucose-sensitive vagal afferents in the liver in comparison with the effect of 2-deoxy-D-glucose. *J. Autonom. Nerv. Syst.* **10**, 255–260.
30. Novin, D., Rogers, R.D., and Hermann, G. (1981). Visceral afferent and efferent connections in the brain. *Diabetologia* **20**, 331–336.
31. Le Magnen, J. (1983). Body energy balance and food intake: a neuroendocrine regulatory mechanism. *Physiol. Rev.* **63**, 314–386.
32. Hauger, R., Hulihan-Giblin, B., Angel, I., Luu, M.D., Janowsky, A., Skolnick, P., and Paul, S.M. (1986). Glucose regulates (^{3}H) (+)-amphetamine binding and Na^+K^+ATPase activity in the hypothalamus: a proposed mechanism for the glucostatic control of feeding and satiety. *Brain Res. Bull.* **16**, 281–288.
33. Rowland, N.E. and Carlton, J. (1986). Neurobiology of an anorectic drug: fenfluramine. *Prog. Neurobiol.* **27**, 13–62.
34. Fisler, J.S. and Bray, G.A. (1985). Dietary obesity: effects of drugs or food intake

in S5B/P1 and Osborne-Mendel rats. *Physiol. Behav.* **34**, 225–231.
35. Bray, G.A., Teague, R.J., and Lee, C.K. (1987). Brain uptake of ketones in rats with differing susceptibility to dietary obesity. *Metabolism* **36**, 27–30.
36. Arase, K., York, D.A., Shargill, N.S., and Bray, G.A. (1987). Effect of cerebroventricular infusions of insulin and beta-hydroxybutyrate on food intake and thermogenesis in the rat. *Clin. Res.* **35**, 767A (Abs).
37. Sakaguchi, T.,Arase, K., and Bray, G.A. (1987b). Effect of intrahypothalamic hydroxybutyrate on sympathetic firing rate. *Metabolism*, **37**, 732–735.
38. Davis, J.D., Wirtshafter, D., Asin, K.E., and Brief, D. (1981). Sustained intracerebroventricular infusion of brain fuels reduces body weight and food intake in rats. *Science* **212**, 81–83.
39. Oku, J., Bray, G.A., Fisler, J.S., and Schemmel, R.A. (1984). Ventromedial hypothalamic knife-cut lesions in rats resistant to dietary obesity. *Am. J. Physiol.* **246**, R943–R948.
40. Schemmel, R.A., Teague, R.J., and Bray, G.A. (1982). Obesity in Osborne-Mendel and S5B/P1 rats: effects of sucrose solutions, castration, and treatment with estradiol or insulin. *Am. J. Physiol.* **243**, R347–R353.
41. Fisler, J.S., Yoshida, T., and Bray, G.A. (1984). Catecholamine turnover in S5B/P1 and Osborne-Mendel rats: response to a high-fat diet. *Am. J. Physiol.* **247**, R290–R295.
42. Bray, G.A., Inoue, S., and Nishizawa, Y. (1981). Hypothalamic obesity. The autonomic hypothesis and the lateral hypothalamus. *Diabetologia* **20**, 366–377.
43. Cox, J.E. and Powley, T.L. (1981). Prior vagotomy blocks VMH obesity in pair-fed rats. *Am. J. Physiol.* **240**, E573–E583.
44. Inoue, S., Mullen, Y.S., and Bray, G.A. (1983). Hyperinsulinemia in rats with hypothalamic obesity. Effects of autonomic drugs and glucose. *Am. J. Physiol.* **245**, R372–R378.
45. Niijima, A., Rohner-Jeanrenaud, F., and Jeanrenaud, B. (1984). Role of ventromedial hypothalamus on sympathetic effects of brown adipose tissue. *Am. J. Physiol.* **247**, R650–R654.
46. Yoshimatsu, H., Niijima, A., Oomura, Y., Kazutoshi, Y., and Katafuchi, T. (1984). Effects of hypothalamic lesion on pancreatic autonomic nerve activity in the rat. *Brain Res.* **303**, 147–152.
47. Nishizawa, Y. and Bray, G.A. (1978). Ventromedial hypothalamic lesions and the mobilization of fatty acids. *J. Clin. Invest.* **61**, 714–721.
48. Young, J.B. and Landsberg, L. (1977b). Suppression of sympathetic nervous system during fasting. *Science* **196**, 1473–1475.
49. Sakaguchi, T. and Bray, G.A. (1987a). The effect of intrahypothalamic injections of glucose on sympathetic effect firing rate. *Brain Res. Bull.* **18**, 591–595.
50. Sakaguchi, T., Takahashi, M., and Bray, G.A. (1986). The diurnal pattern of food intake is controlled by the suprachiasmatic nucleus (SCN). *Clin. Res.* **34**, 553A (Abs).
51. Young, J.B., Saville, E., Rothwell, N.J., Stock, M.J., and Landsberg, L. (1982).

Effect of diet and cold exposure on norepinephrine turnover in brown adipose tissue of the rat. *J. Clin. Invest.* **69**, 1061–1071.
52. Yoshida, T., Kemnitz, J.W., and Bray, G.A. (1983). Lateral hypothalamic lesions and norepinephrine turnover in rats. *J. Clin. Invest.* **72**, 919–927.
53. Van Itallie, T.B. and Kissileff, H.R. (1985). Physiology of food intake: an inventory control model. *Am. J. Clin. Nutr.* **42**, 914–923.
54. Young, J.B. and Landsberg, L. (1977a). Stimulation of the sympathetic nervous system during sucrose feeding. Nature **269**, 615–617.
55. Bray, G.A. (1982). Regulation of energy balance: studies on genetic, hypothalamic and dietary obesity. *Proc. Nutr. Soc.* **41**, 95–108.
56. Bruce, B.K., King, B.M., Phelps, G.R., and Veitia, M.C. (1982). Effects of adrenalectomy and corticosterone administration on hypothalamic obesity in rats. *Am. J. Physiol.* **243**, E152–E157.
57. Mook, D.G., Kenney, N.J., Roberts, S., Nussbaum, A.I., and Rodier, W.I., III (1982). Ovarianadrenal interactions in regulation of body weight by female rats. *J. Comp. Physiol. Psychol.* **81**, 198–211.
58. Bray, G.A. (1986). Autonomic and endocrine factors in the regulation of energy balance. *Fed. Proc.* **45**, 1404–1410.
59. Bray, G.A. (1984). Integration of energy intake and expenditure in animals and man: the autonomic and adrenal hypothesis. *Clin. Endocrinol. Metab.* **13**, 521–546.
60. Sato, M. and Bray, G.A. (1984). Adrenalectomy and food restriction in the genetically obese (*ob/ob*) mouse. *Am. J. Physiol.* **246**, R20–R25.
61. Holt, S. and York, D.A. (1982). The effect of adrenalectomy on GDP binding to brown adipose tissue mitochondria of obese rats. *Biochem. J.* **208**, 819–822.
62. Marchington, D., Rothwell, N.J., Stock, M.J., and York, D.A. (1983). Energy balance, diet-induced thermogenesis and brown adipose tissue in lean and obese (*fa/fa*) Zucker rats after adrenalectomy. *J. Nutr.* **113**, 1395–1402.
63. Fukushima, M., Lupien, J., and Bray, G.A. (1985). Interaction of light and corticosterone on food intake and interscapular brown adipose tissue of rats. *Am. J. Physiol.* **249**, R753–R757.
64. vander Tuig, J.G., Ohshima, K., Yoshida, T., Romsos, D.R., and Bray, G.A. (1984). Adrenalectomy increases norepinephrine turnover in brown adipose tissue of obese (*ob/ob*) mice. *Life Sci.* **31**, 1423–1432.
65. York, D.A., Marchington, D., Holt, S.J., and Allars, J. (1985). Regulation of sympathetic activity in lean and obese Zucker rats. *Am. J. Physiol.* **249**, E299–E305.
66. Levine, A.S., Rogers, B., Kneip, J., Grace, M., and Morley, J.E. (1983). Effect of centrally administered corticotropin-releasing factor (CRF) on multiple feeding paradigms. *Neuropharmacology* **22**, 337–339.
67. Morley, J.E., Levine, A.S., and Rowland, N.E. (1983). Stress induced eating. *Life Sci.* **32**, 2169–2182.

68. Brown, M.R., Fisher, L.A., Rivier, J., Spiess, J., Rivier, C., and Vale, W. (1982). Corticotropin releasing factor: actions on the sympathetic nervous system and metabolism. *Endocrinology* **111**, 928-931.

Diet and Obesity, Bray, G.A. et al., eds., pp. 37-50.
Japan Sci. Soc. Press, Tokyo/S. Karger, Basel (1988)

Hormonal Regulation of Appetite and Fat Accumulation in Obesity

SHUJI INOUE, SHINOBU SATOH, AND
MASATO EGAWA

The Third Department of Internal Medicine, Yokohama City University, Yokohama 232, Japan

There are two hormones which clearly stimulate appetite and fat accumulation in animals : insulin and corticosterone. In this paper we will emphasize the importance of insulin in the development of obesity referring to the pathogenesis of ventromedial hypothalamic (VMH) obesity.

VMH obesity is produced by destruction of the ventromedial region of the hypothalamus. This obesity has been recognized for more than 75 years and was defined experimentally by Hetherington and Ranson in 1940 (*1*). VMH obesity is associated with a number of changes of which hyperphagia and increased concentrations of insulin are supposed to be most important in its development (*2*).

I. IMPORTANCE OF HYPERINSULINEMIA IN THE DEVELOPMENT OF OBESITY

Brobeck found hyperphagia in VMH obesity in 1960 (3). In the many years since then, the pathogenesis of VMH obesity has been considered to be due to the destruction of a "satiety center" in the ventromedial hypothalamus. Ablation of this "satiety center"was believed to remove the inhibitory influences to a "hunger center" in the lateral hypothalamus and allow excess feeding. This excessive amount of food intake made animals obese (*3*).

Several investigations have suggested that this interpretation may be incorrect. Han and Liu demonstrated that VMH lesioned rats manifest obesity even if hyperphagia is prevented by force feeding (*4*).

When increased concentrations of insulin were first reported in VMH obesity, the hyperinsulinemia was presumed to be secondary to hyperphagia, since the former disappeared after long fasting. But it was demonstrated that restricted feeding or pair-feeding failed to eliminate the hyperinsulinemia (*5, 6*). This condition occurs within minutes or in the first few days after ventromedial hypothalamic lesions even without hyperphagia or obesity (*6–8*). York and Bray (*9*) and Goldman et al. (*10*) demonstrated that when β-cells of the pancreas were destroyed beforehand with streptozotocin to prevent the increase of insulin after VMH lesions, obesity and hyperphagia were prevented or remarkably attenuated.

Since insulin treatment can produce hyperphagia and obesity, the focus of attention gradually shifted to the hyperinsulinemia. However, the question remained unsettled as to whether hyperphagia or hyperinsulinemia was the primary factor in the development of hypothalamic obesity in the 1970s. The mechanism for the increase of insulin in VMH obesity also remained to be settled. It is not secondary to the hyperphagia or obesity because hyperinsulinemia occurs even when the food intake is limited and the increase of body weight is prevented (*5–7*). Two hypotheses have been advanced. One is humoral, postulating that a "hypothalamic factor" which stimulates or suppresses pancreatic β-cells is released into the circulation from the hypothalamus and thus increases release of insulin (*11, 12*). The other hypothesis proposes "neural mediation" which implies that stimuli for increased release of insulin by the β- cells occurs through the autonomic nervous system (*13*).

To clarify these questions, we performed the following experi-

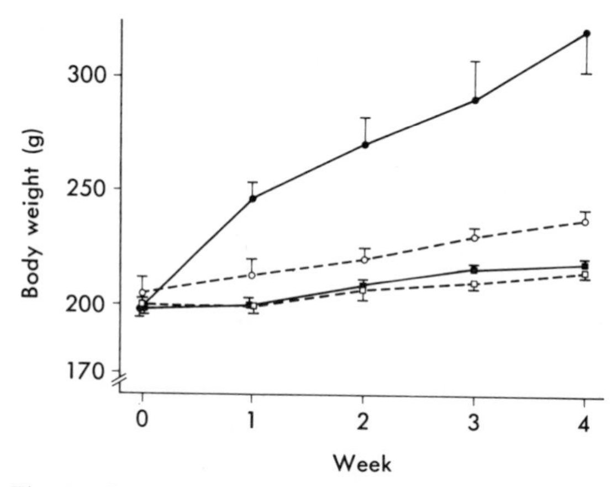

Fig. 1. Body weight of VMH lesioned and sham lesioned rats. Each group is plotted as mean±S.E. N, intact pancreas; T, pancreatic transplants; ● N-VMH; ○ T-VMH; ■ N-sham-VMH; ○ T-sham-VMH.

TABLE I
Effects of VMH Lesions on Body Fatness and Food Intake

Group	Body density[a]	Lee Index[a]	Food intake[b] (g/day)
VMH intact pancreas	1.0253±0.0167	0.327±0.004	29.8±0.8
Sham intact pancreas	1.0770±0.0030	0.288±0.002	17.1±0.4
VMH pancreatic transplants	1.0654±0.0116	0.296±0.002	20.5±0.5
Sham pancreatic transplants	1.0794±0.0046	0.292±0.003	16.7±0.4

Values are means±S.E. Lee Index = $\sqrt[3]{\text{body wt}}$ (g)/length (cm).
[a]Data were obtained 4 weeks after VMH lesions.
[b]Data were obtained during 2nd week.

ment (*14, 15*). In inbred Lewis rats, pancreatic β-cells were destroyed by treatment with streptozoticin. Subsequently, several fetal pancreases were transplanted underneath the renal capsule. In this

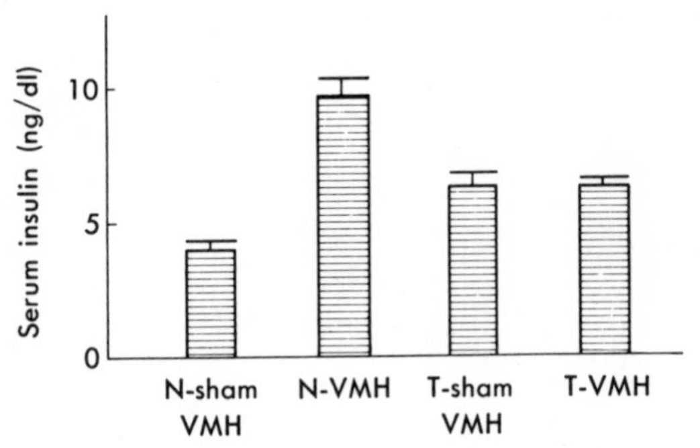

Fig. 2. Serum insulin in VMH lesioned and sham lesioned rats. N, intact pancreas; T, pancreatic transplants. Modified from ref. *15*.

way we could have rats with denervated pancreatic tissue. After recovery from diabetes, VMH lesions were performed and the rats were observed for 4 weeks.

VMH lesioned rats with an intact pancreas gained weight rapidly after VMH lesions, showing typical weight gain of dynamic phase (Fig. 1). VMH lesioned rats with pancreatic transplants gained slowly, showing the same level of weight gain as non lesioned control rats. Body fatness was compared by the methods of body density and Lee Index. VMH lesioned rats with an intact pancreas were fatter than non lesioned control rats in both comparisons, while VMH lesioned rats with pancreatic transplants were not (Table I).

VMH lesioned rats with an intact pancreas had serum insulin levels increased about 3-fold over non lesioned control rats with intact pancreatic tissue, whereas VMH lesioned rats with pancreatic transplants showed the same insulin levels as non lesioned rats with pancreatic transplants (Fig. 2). The differences in serum insulin levels between control rats with an intact pancreas and those with pancreatic transplants may be explained by the fact that insulin is released into circulation and does not immediately traverse the liver in the rats with pancreatic transplants (*16*).

VMH lesioned rats with an intact pancreas increased food

intake by 70%, whereas VMH lesioned rats with pancreatic transplants increased it by 20% when hyperinsulinemia was prevented (Table I). If a humoral factor were the stimulus to pancreatic β-cells, this factor should reach the pancreatic tissue underneath the renal capsule and should have increased insulin release. Our results supported the hypothesis that the hyperinsulinemia of VMH obesity is neurally mediated and is most important for the development of VMH obesity.

II. NEURAL COMPONENTS OF HYPERINSULINEMIA

Both the sympathetic and parasympathetic nervous system appear to be involved in the hyperinsulinemia of VMH lesioned rats. Evidence for vagal hyperactivity came first from measurement of gastric acid. Ridley and Brooks demonstrated that VMH lesioned rats had gastric hyperacidity, a phenomenon related to vagal overactivity (*17*). This result was subsequently confirmed by Powley and Opsahl (*18*) and by Inoue and Bray (*19*). In 1974 Powley and Opsahl demonstrated that interruption of the vagus nerves below the diaphragm could reverse the obesity which follows VMH lesions (*18*). They suggested that hypersecretion of insulin was reduced after vagotomy and that reversal of obesity occurred because the hyperinsulinemia was removed. We repeated this study and found that the reversal of body weight after subdiaphragmatic vagotomy was due to restriction of food intake secondary to slowed gastric emptying (*19*). Nevertheless, we found a positive correlation between serum insulin and gastric acidity in VMH lesioned rats in the same experiment. Berthoud and Jeanrenaud reported that acute hyperinsulinemia, which started within an hour after VMH lesions, could be reversed by acute vagotomy (*20*). These findings suggest that the stimulatory effect of vagus contributes to the hyperinsulinemia in VMH lesioned rats (*2*).

The sympathetic nervous system appears to be less active after VMH lesions. This is indicated by the findings of smaller submaxillary salivary glands with reduced serum glucagon levels, impaired fat mobilization after various stresses and reduced β-hydroxylase

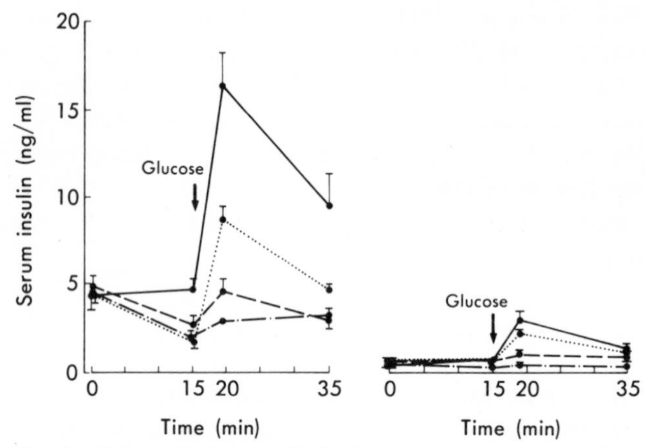

Fig. 3. Effects of pharmacological agents on serum insulin in VMH lesioned (left) and sham lesioned (right) rats. Infusions lasted throughout the experiment and bolus injection of glucose was given at 15 min ●—● saline; ●- -● epinephrine; ●···● atropine; ●-·-● epinephrine +atropine. Modified from ref. *25*.

release into the circulation (*21–23*). This factor can contribute to the hyperinsulinemia after VMH lesions (*24*).

In order to explore more thoroughly the relative contribution of each component of the autonomic nervous system to this hyperinsulinemia, we performed the following experiments (*25*). Four weeks after VMH lesions, rats which had been fasted overnight were infused with epinephrine (1.0 μg/min/kg) to remove the effects of the sympathetic nervous system. Firing of the vagus was inhibited by administration of atropine (1 mg/kg intraperitoneally and 1 mg/kg subcutaneously).

When epinephrine was infused, basal insulin levels decreased and glucose-induced insulin secretion was inhibited by 83% in VMH lesioned rats (Fig. 3). When atropine was given, it also significantly decreased basal insulin levels and inhibited glucose-induced insulin secretion by 42% in VMH lesioned rats. When the effects of epinephrine and atropine were combined, basal insulin levels became markedly decreased and glucose-induced insulin secretion was completely inhibited in VMH lesioned rats. In normal rats, similar

TABLE II
Serum Insulin Levels in Response to Oral Glucose Load (lg/kg)

Group	0 min	30 min (peak)
VMH	3.10±0.93	5.04±1.16
VMH+vagotomy	1.80±0.51**	3.34±0.67**
Sham-operated (control)	0.49±0.07	1.03±0.17

**$p<0.01$.

results were observed, but to a much lesser extent than in VMH lesioned rats.

To further investigate the role of vagus nerve on hyperinsulinemia after VMH lesions, the effect of selective vagotomy of the pancreatic branch was examined. The selective vagotomy was done 3 weeks after VMH lesions using microsurgery technique.

During oral glucose tolerance tests, selective vagotomy decreased basal insulin by 42% and inhibited glucose-induced insulin secretion at peak value by 34% in VMH lesioned rats (Table II). In contrast, no significant effect was observed in control rats.

It is also important to note that selective vagotomy did not completely restore insulin secretion to normal in VMH lesioned rats.

These two results suggest that stimulation of the vagus nerve and suppression of sympathetic nerves both contribute to the hyperinsulinemia that follows VMH lesions.

III. HYPERINSULINEMIA AND FAT ACCUMULATION

Obesity is a consequence of excessive fat accumulation. Three factors can contribute to this process, (1) increased lipogenesis in the liver and adipose tissue, (2) increased fat deposition in the adipose tissue, and (3) reduced lipolysis from the adipose tissue.

As to hepatic lipogenesis in the liver, triglyceride secretion rate from the liver and serum insulin was measured (*26*). There was a significant increase in triglyceride secretion rate and serum insulin in VMH lesioned rats, revealing a positive correlation between them (Fig. 4). To assess lipogenic capacity in the adipose tissue, the activity of a key lipogenic enzyme, pyruvate dehydrogenase and

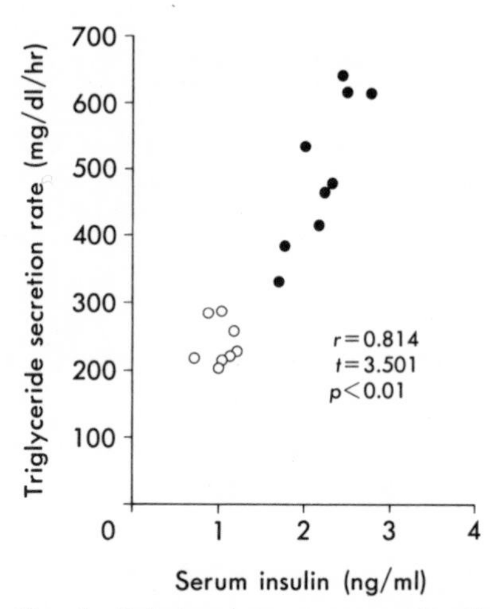

Fig. 4 Relation between serum insulin and triglyceride secretion rate from the liver in VMH lesioned (●) and sham lesioned (○) rats ($r=0.81$, $p<0.01$) Modified from ref. *26*.

serum insulin were determined (*27*). VMH lesioned rats showed significantly increased pyruvate dehydrogenase activity and serum insulin in the fed state, which decreased significantly after 48 hr of fasting; there was a positive correlation between the two factors (Fig. 5).

To investigate fat deposition into the adipose tissue, heparin releasable lipoprotein lipase activity and insulin in the blood of fed rats was measured (*28*). VMH lesioned rats showed significantly increased lipoprotein lipase activity and serum insulin; there was a positive correlation between them (Fig. 6).

To investigate lipolysis in adipose tissue, glycerol release and serum insulin were determined. Under basal conditions, there was no difference in glycerol release between VMH lesioned and control rats (Fig. 7). VMH lesioned rats showed significantly lower glycerol release in response to epinephrine and isoproterenol, but higher serum insulin levels. There was a negative correlation between serum insulin and epinephrine induced glycerol release ($r=-0.76$, $p<0.02$).

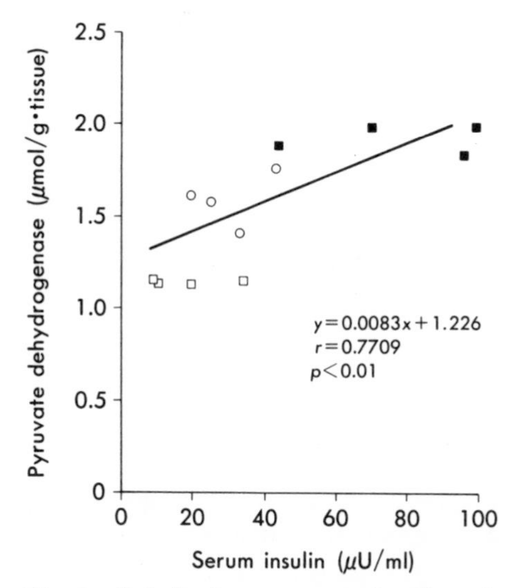

Fig. 5. Relation between serum insulin and pyruvate dehydrogenase activity in the adipose tissue ($r=0.82$, $p<0.02$). ■ VMH lesioned rats (*ad lib*); □ VMH lesioned rats (48 hr fasting); ○ sham lesioned rats (*ad lib*).

These results indicate that hyperinsulinemia after VMH lesions contributes to excessive fat accumulation.

IV. HYPERINSULINEMIA AND HYPERPHAGIA

With hyperinsulinemia, food intake increased by 70% after VMH lesions, whereas without hyperinsulinemia, it increased by only 20% in the experiment with pancreatic transplantation (*14, 15*). This suggests that hyperphagia in VMH lesioned rats is due in part to the hyperinsulinemia.

The mechanism of hyperphagia produced by hyperinsulinemia is unknown and requires further investigation. Several possibilities can be postulated: (1) increasing peripheral glucose utilization produced by hyperinsulinemia could serve as a signal for food-seeking behavior, although hyperphagia in response to real hypoglycemia produced by hyperinsulinemia has been denied (*29*); (2)

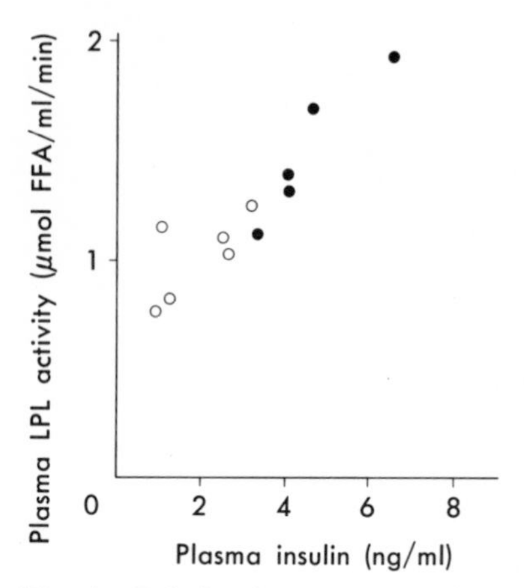

Fig. 6. Relation between serum insulin and plasma lipoprotein lipase activity in VMH lesioned (●) and sham lesioned (○) rats ($r = 0.95$, $p < 0.02$) Modified from ref. *28*.

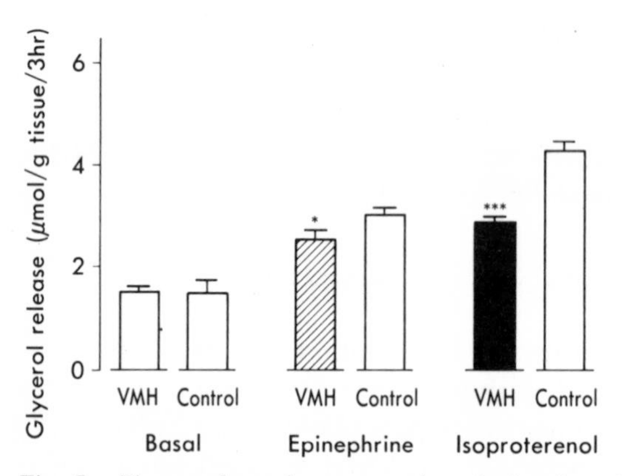

Fig. 7. Plasma glycerol concentrations in basal, and after epinephrine and isoprotelenol stimulation. $*p < 0.05$, $**p < 0.001$.

glucoprivation by insulin in cerebral glucoreceptor cells could also stimulate food intake (*30*); (3) insulin receptors in the nuclei of the lateral hypothalamus, as proposed by Oomura and Kita (*31*), could explain the mechanism of hyperphagia by hyperinsulinemia; and (4)

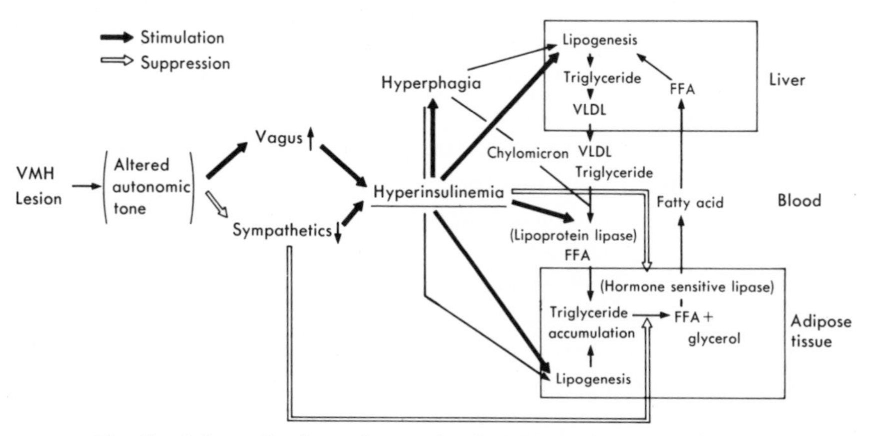

Fig. 8. Schema for the pathogenesis of VMH obesity (see text).

hyperinsulinemia may have a close relationship to peptide hormones which stimulate or inhibit food intake such as cholecystokinin or β-endorphin.

SUMMARY

This paper has developed an autonomic hypothesis for explaining the metabolic features which occur after VMH lesions (*32*). This hypothesis could also explain the mechanisms for development of VMH obesity in a framework like that shown in Fig. 8.

VMH lesions would produce derangements of the autonomic nervous system, suppressing the sympathetic nerves and stimulating the vagus. The combined effects would produce hyperinsulinemia.

The hyperinsulinemia would increase lipogenesis in liver and adipose tissue, increase lipoprotein lipase activity resulting in acceleration of deposition of exogenous (chylomicron) and endogenous (very low density lipoprotein (VLDL) triglyceride) lipids into adipose tissue and reduce lipolysis in adipose tissue.

Hyperphagia which is produced by hyperinsulinemia would provide excessive foodstuffs for lipogenesis and chylomicrons for fat deposition. All of these effects cooperatively work for excessive fat accumulation and contribute to the development of VMH obesity.

Recently, reports have appeared which propose corticosterone may be the primary factor in the development of ventromedial hypothalamic obesity (*33, 34*).

Adrenalectomy could reverse the obesity (*33, 34*). However, King and Smith (*35*) noted that: 1) hypophysectomy or incomplete adrenalectomy should have also reduced the development of obesity, and 2) only a small amount of corticosterone replacement was enough for the development of obesity in complete adrenalectomized rats with VMH lesions. Based on these results, they interpreted that the role of corticosterone is permissive or indirect and not direct in the development of VMH obesity.

REFERENCES

1. Hetherington, A. and Ranson, S.W. (1940). Hypothalamic lesions and adiposity in the rat. *Anat. Rec.* **78**, 149-172.
2. Bray, G.A. and York, D.A. (1979). Hypothalamic and genetic obesity in experimental animals: An autonomic and endocrine hypothesis. *Physiol. Rev.* **59**, 718-809.

3a. Brobeck, J.R. (1946). Mechanism of development of obesity in animals with hypothalamic lesions. *Physiol. Rev.* **26**, 541-559.

3b. Brobeck, J.R. (1960) Food and temperature. *Recent Prog. Horm. Res.* **16**, 439-466.

4. Han, P.W. and Liu, A.C. (1966). Obesity and impaired growth of rats force-fed 40 days after hypothalamic lesions. *Am. J. Physiol.* **211**, 229-231.
5. Han, P.W. and Frohman, L.A. (1970). Hyperinsulinemia in tube-fed hypophysectomized rats bearing hypothalamic lesions. *Am. J. Physiol.* **219**, 1632-1636.
6. Hustvedt, B.E. and Løvø, A. (1972). Correlation between hyperinsulinemia and hyperphagia in rats with ventromedial hypothalamic lesions. *Acta Physiol. Scand.* **84**, 29-33.
7. Martin, J. M., Konijnendijk, W., and Bouman, P.R. (1974). Insulin and growth hormone secretion in rats with ventromedial hypothalamic lesions maintained on restricted food intake. *Diabetes* **23**, 203-208.
8. Rohner, F., Dufour, A.C., Karakash, C., Marchand, Y.L., Ruf, K.B., and Jeanrenaud. B. (1977). Immediate effect of lesion of the ventromedial hypothalamic area upon glucose-induced insulin secretion in anaesthetized rats. *Diabetologia* **13**, 239-242.
9. York, D.A. and Bray, G.A. (1972). Dependence of hypothalamic obesity on insulin, the pituitary and the adrenal gland. *Endocrinology* **90**, 885-894.

10. Goldman, J.K., Schnatz, J.D., Bernardis, L.L., and Frohman, L.A. (1972). Effects of ventromedial hypothalamic destruction in rats with pre-existing streptozotocin induced diabetes. *Metabolism* **21**, 132-136.
11. Lockhart-Ewart, R. B., Mok, C., and Martin, J.M. (1976). Neuroendocrine control of insulin secretion. *Diabetes* **25**, 96-100.
12. Moltz, J.H., Dobbs, R.E., McCann, S.M., and Fawcett, C.P. (1977). Effects of hypothalamic factors on insulin and glucagon release from the islets of Langerhans. *Endocrinology* **101**, 196-202.
13. Bernardis, L.L. and Frohman, L.A. (1970). Effect of lesion size in the ventromedial hypothalamus on growth hormone and insulin levels in the weanling rat. *Neuroendocrinology* **6**, 319-328.
14. Inoue, S., Bray, G.A., and Mullen, Y.S. (1977). Effect of transplantation of pancreas on development of hypothalamic obesity. *Nature* **266**, 742-744.
15. Inoue, S., Bray, G.A., and Mullen, Y.S. (1978). Transplantation of pancreatic β-cells prevents development of hypothalamic obesity in rats. *Am. J. Physiol.* **235**, E266-E271.
16. Weber, C. J., Hardy, M.A., Lerner, R.L., Felig, P., and Reemtsma, K. (1976). Hyperinsulinemia and hyperglucagonemia following pancreatic islet transplantation in diabetic rats. *Diabetes* **25**, 944-948.
17. Ridley, P.T. and Brooks, F.P. (1965). Alterations in gastric secretion following hypothalamic lesions producing hyperphagia. *Am. J. Physiol.* **209**, 319-323.
18. Powley, T.L. and Opsahl, C.A. (1974) Ventromedial hypothalamic obesity abolished by subdiaphragmatic vagotomy. *Am. J. Physiol.* **226**, 25-33.
19. Inoue, S. and Bray, G.A. (1977). The effects of subdiaphragmatic vagotomy in rats with ventromedial hypothalamic obesity. *Endocrinology* **100**, 108-114.
20. Berthoud, H.R. and Jeanrenaud, B. (1979). Acute hyperinsulinemia and its reversal by vagotomy after lesions of the ventromedial hypothalamus in anesthetized rats. *Endocrinology* **105**, 146-151.
21. Inoue, S., Campfield, L.A., and Bray, G.A. (1977). Comparison of metabolic alterations in hypothalamic and high fat diet-induced obesity. *Am. J. Physiol.* **233**, R162-R168.
22. Nishizawa, Y. and Bray, G.A. (1978). Ventromedial hypothalamic lesions and the mobilization of fatty acids. *J. Clin. Invest.* **61**, 714-721.
23. Inoue, S. and Bray, G.A.(1980). Role of the autonomic nervous system in the development of ventromedial hypothalamic obesity. *Brain Res. Bull.* **5** (Suppl. 4), 119-125.
24. Woods, S.C. and Porte, D., Jr. (1974) Neural control of the endocrine pancreas. *Physiol. Rev.* **54**, 596-619.
25. Inoue, S., Mullen, Y.S., and Bray, G.A. (1983). Hyperinsulinaemia in rats with hypothalamic obesity: effects of autonomic drugs and glucose. *Am. J. Physiol.* **245**, R372-R378.
26. Satoh, S., Inoue, S., Egawa, M., Takamura, Y., and Murase, T. (1985). Increased triglyceride secretion rate and hyperinsulinemia in ventromedial hypothalamic

lesioned rats *in vivo*. *Acta Endocrinol.* **100**, 6-9.

27. Inoue, S. and Bray G.A. (1981). Ventromedial hypothalamic obesity and autonomic nervous system: An autonomic hypothesis. *In* "The Body Weight Regulatory System: Normal and Disturbed Mechanisms," Cioffi, L.A. *et al*., eds., pp. 61-64, Raven Press, New York.
28. Inoue, S. and Murase, T. (1982). Increase of postheparin plasma-lipoprotein-lipase activity in ventromedial hypothalamic obesity in rats. *Int. J. Obesity* **6**, 259-266.
29. Bray, G.A. and Gallagher, T.F., Jr. (1975). Manifestations of hypothalamic obesity in man : A comprehensive investigation of eight patients and a review of the literature. *Medicine* **54**, 301-330.
30. Smith, G. and Epstein, A. (1969). Increased feeding in response to decreased utilization in the rat and monkey. *Am. J. Physiol.* **217**, 1083-1087.
31. Oomura, Y. and Kita, H. (1981). Insulin acting as a modulator of feeding through the hypothalamus. *Diabetologia* **20** (Suppl.), 290-298.
32. Inoue, S. and Bray, G.A. (1979). An autonomic hypothesis for hypothalamic obesity. *Life Sci.* **25**, 561-566.
33. Debons, A.F., Zurek, L.D., Tse, C.S., and Abrahamsen, S. (1986). Central nervous system control of hyperphagia in hypothalamic obesity: Dependence on adrenal glucocorticoids. *Endocrinology* **118**, 1678-1681.
34. King, B.M., Calvert, C.B., Esquerre, K.R., Kaufman, J.H., and Frohman, L.A. (1984). Relation between plasma corticosterone and insulin levels in rats with ventromedial hypothalamic lesions. *Physiol. Behav.* **32**, 991-994.
35. King, B.M. and Smith, R.L. (1985). Hypothalamic obesity after hypophysectomy or adrenalectomy : dependence on corticosterone. *Am. J. Physiol.* **249**, R522-R526.

Diet and Obesity, Bray, G.A. et al., eds., pp. 51–60.
Japan Sci. Soc. Press, Tokyo/S. Karger, Basel (1988)

Physiological Regulation of Intakes of Carbohydrate, Fat, and Protein

JUDITH S. STERN,[*1,*2] THOMAS W. CASTONGUAY,[*1,*4] AND QUINTON R. ROGERS[*3,*4]

*Department of Nutrition,[*1] Division of Clinical Nutrition in the Department of Internal Medicine,[*2] Department of Physiological Sciences,[*3] and The Food Intake Laboratory,[*4] University of California, Davis, California 95616, U.S.A.*

The factors that influence food intake and food selection are both numerous and complex (for reviews *1–3*). These include physiological and metabolic factors such as the hormonal milieu, neurotransmitter levels in the brain, and the presence of certain diseases. In addition, the choice of food is influenced by hedonic (palatability, taste, texture, odor, appearance), social (religion, culture), and environmental (temperature) factors. The selection of food can also be modified by drugs, specific appetites, and by learned preferences and aversions. In this chapter, we will review some of the physiological factors involved in influencing the choice of macronutrients—protein, carbohydrate, and fat.

While early studies showing diet selection did not use "pure" macronutrient sources, they did demonstrate that dietary choice of animals from a number of different species was sensitive to the nutritional composition of the diet. These studies showed that some animals could "self select" a nutritionally adequate diet from a variety of nutrient sources (*4*). In 1915, for example, Evvard demonstrated that pigs could compose an adequate diet from several different food sources (*5*). Three years later, Osborne and Mendel reported that laboratory rats selected diets that were nutritionally adequate in preference to similar but protein-deficient diets (*6*). A classic 1928 report in human infants revealed that they too could select a diet that appeared to meet both caloric and nutrient requirements (*7*). While this later study has been criticized because the food items available were mostly adequate by themselves, Davis' work was a catalyst to future work in this area. Finally, at about the same time, Richter demonstrated that, in rats, the selection of food was influenced by bodily need (*8*). Pancreatectomized rats, for example, decrease their intake of carbohydrate and increase their intake of fat in order to maintain blood glucose homeostasis (*9*).

I. PROTEIN

The quality or the amino acid composition of a protein has a large influence on selection and intake. To quote from a review by Gietzen and her colleagues (*10*): there are three typical responses of rats to diets which vary in amount and quality of amino acids:

1. Rats will eat a diet within a certain range (20–30%) of protein levels without altering their food intake.
2. Rats will eat less of a diet that is very high or very low in protein.
3. Rats will dramatically decrease their food intake when presented with a diet that is devoid of or that has an excess of one essential amino acid.

What is the critical event that signals brain centers to have the animal select protein? It has been proposed that the signal includes the concentration of circulating tryptophan (the essential amino acid precursor for the synthesis of brain serotonin) and its proportion to the neutral amino acid with which tryptophan competes to cross the blood-brain barrier (*11*). Peters and Harper have challenged the tryptophan/serotonin hypothesis (*12*). They do not observe a consistent correlation between protein consumption and either the ratio of plasma tryptophan:neutral amino acids or brain serotonin concentration. Other researchers have suggested that

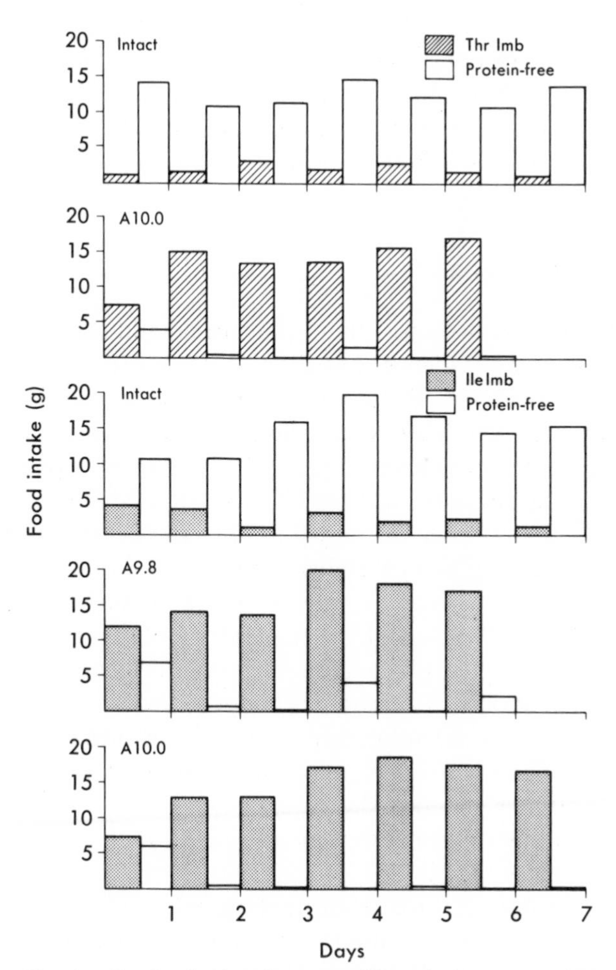

Fig. 1. Food selection by prepyriform lesioned rats fed threonine (Thr) imbalanced or iso-leucine (Ile) imbalanced and protein-free diets. From ref. *14*.

protein consumption is under dopaminergic control (*13*).

While the metabolic signal is not known, the prepyriform cortex in the brain appears to be involved in the response of the rat to an amino acid imbalanced diet (*14*). Within 30 min of being given an amino acid imbalanced diet, a hungry rat dramatically decreases its food intake. Electrolytic lesions in the prepyriform cortex attenuate the response of the rat to an amino acid imbalanced diet. When given a choice between either a threonine or iso-leucine imbalanced diet and a protein-free diet, rats select the protein-free diet (see Fig. 1, ref. *14*). Prepyriform cortex lesions abolish this effect.

II. FAT AND CARBOHYDRATE

Less is known about factors that influence fat and carbohydrate intake. There is some evidence that disease states can alter carbohydrate and fat selection. Rats, when treated with insulin, will selectively increase carbohydrate consumption (*15*). However, depending on the severity of diabetes, rats will either select a relatively high fat diet (mild streptozotocin (STZ) diabetes, 35 mg/kg body weight) or a relatively high carbohydrate diet (moderate to severe STZ diabetes, 65 mg/kg body weight) (*16*).

There is much debate as to whether some obese humans are "carbohydrate cravers." Some of the research of Wurtman and her colleagues has shown that obese subjects, who crave carbohydrate, will decrease their intake of "carbohydrate-rich" snacks in response to the administration of d-fenfluramine (*17*). This would imply that brain serotonin was involved in monitoring carbohydrate intake. This interpretation is tenuous, however, since many of these so-called "carbohydrate-rich" snacks were also high in fat. Some of the foods had a greater percentage of calories from fat than from carbohydrate (*e.g.*, donuts, ice cream, potato chips).

It may be that obese individuals prefer the combination of high sugar and high fat foods. Work by Drewnowski has shown that when asked to rate dairy products with varying amounts of fat and sugar, reduced obese individuals prefer sweetened, high fat dairy products (*18*). If these preferences are ultimately reflected in excess daily intake, the excessive consumption of these foods could contribute to weight regain. Suzuki has reported that when rats eat the combination of sugar and fat, they get fatter than do rats that are fed the same amounts of sugar and fat, but in separate meals (*19*).

Suzuki has speculated that this occurs because sugar stimulates insulin release which then increases the activity of adipose tissue lipoprotein lipase. Circulating triglycerides can then readily be stored in adipose tissue.

Our work in experimental animals is supportive of the observation that obese individuals prefer fat. When the genetically obese Zucker rat (*fafa*) is allowed to compose a diet from protein, carbohydrate, and fat, they "self-select" a diet high in fat, with over 60% of calories from fat (*20, 21*). In contrast, genetically lean rats (*Fa/?*) self-select a diet lower in fat (less than 40% of calories from fat) and higher in carbohydrate. Adrenal glucocorticoids are associated with this phenomenon. Adrenalectomy decreases and normalizes food intake and fat selection by the obese rat (Figs. 2 and 3). In addition, weight and fat gain, plasma insulin levels and activity of adipose tissue lipoprotein lipase are decreased (*21*).

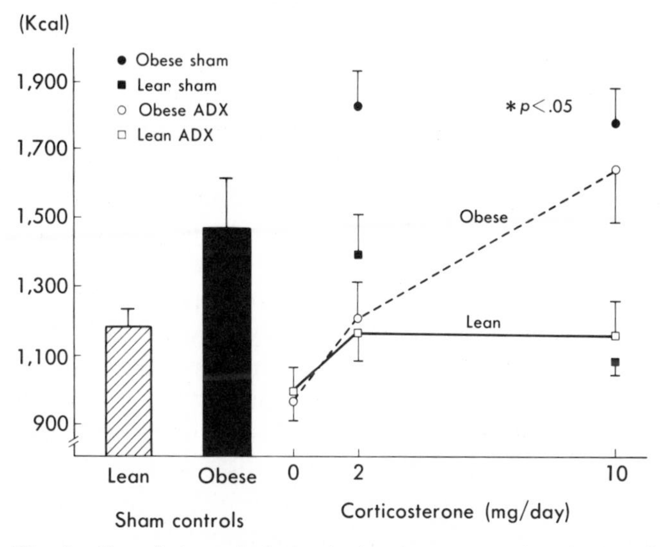

Fig. 2. Cumulative caloric intake by sham-operated and adrenalectomized (ADX), female obese and lean Zucker rats given one of three doses of corticosterone (0, 2 mg or 10 mg/day) for 17 days. Adrenalectomies were performed at 11 weeks of age. From ref. *21*.

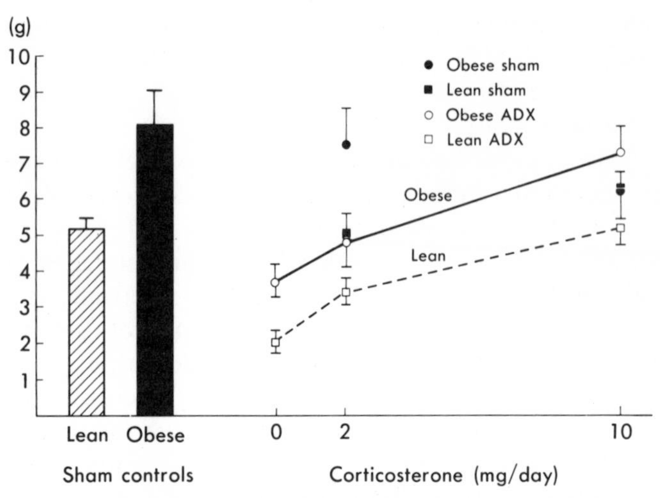

Fig. 3. Daily average fat intake by sham-operated and adrenalectomized (ADX), female obese and lean Zucker rats given one of three doses of corticosterone (0, 2 mg or 10 mg/day) for 17 days. Rats were 11 weeks of age when they were adrenalectomized. From ref. *21*.

Corticosterone therapy, applied to adrenalectomized rats, restores fat selection and total daily food intake to pre-operative levels in a dose-dependent fashion (see Figs. 2 and 3). Corticosterone-replaced, adrenalectomized obese Zucker rats also resume their characteristically high rate of weight and fat gain. While the precise mechanism governing fat selection in the genetically obese rat is not known, it is possible that adrenocorticotropic hormone (ACTH) or corticotropin releasing hormone (CRH) may be involved (*21*).

Other studies of dietary selection patterns of adrenalectomized Sprague-Dawley rats have emphasized some of the changes that are observed in carbohydrate choice (*13*). Recent work by Romsos and his colleagues has suggested that the discrepancies in selection patterns between the two rat strains may be accounted for in the composition of the dietary macronutrient sources (*22*). They have convincingly shown that the composition of the carbohydrate fraction (either glucose or starch based) can be effective in altering the appetitive response of adrenalectomized genetically obese (*ob/ob*)

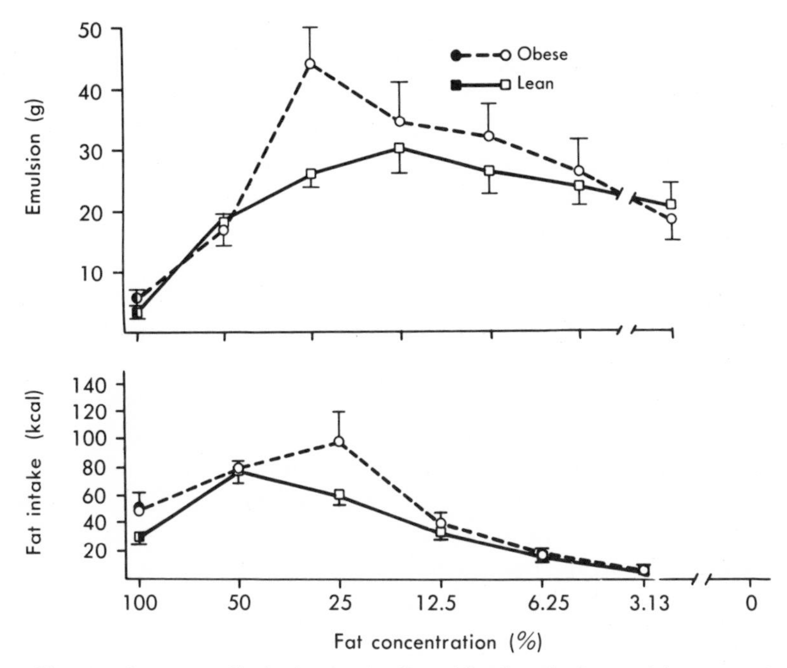

Fig. 4. Average daily fat intake (kcal) and intake of a fat emulsion (grams) by 10-week old, female obese and lean Zucker rats given access to protein, carbohydrate and fat. The fat source (corn oil) was diluted with water by adding an emulsifier (0.5% sodium stearoyl-2-lactylate) to the corn oil/water mixture. From ref. *23*.

mice. Mice given complex carbohydrate typically reduce consumption and lose weight. Adrenalectomized obese mice given access to diets that have a high percentage of glucose do not typically reduce intake or rate of weight gain. These results suggest that adrenalectomy may be effective in altering carbohydrate selection under a narrow range of dietary conditions. Further research along these lines would contribute significantly in developing our understanding of some of the factors that permit the selecting animal to trade off calories derived from dietary fat and carbohydrate sources.

In addition to dietary factors altering intake, sensory qualities and caloric density can alter selection, especially for fat. For example, when obese and lean Zucker rats are given access to three macronutrient sources, and the fat source is corn oil, both groups avidly drink enough corn oil to have it represent from 30 to 50% of their total daily caloric intake (*23, 24*). When the fat source (100% corn oil) is diluted (by the addition of an emulsifier and water), "fat appetite" is promoted in both lean and obese rats (*23*). Within a wide range of concentrations, both obese and lean rats will compensate for dilution by increasing their intake of diluted fat (see Fig. 4). Under some conditions, the compensation for the dilution results in greater dietary fat intake than had been found under original conditions.

Although it was thought that the increase in intake of diluted sugar solutions reflected changes in the palatability of the solution, further analysis has led to the conclusion that at least within a wide range of concentrations rats will attempt to compensate for dilution by increasing intake so as to preserve a fixed proportion of their total intake from their carbohydrate source (*25*). Whether or not dietary fat is similarly defended requires further research.

SUMMARY

Evidence is presented that an animal's selection of protein, fat, and carbohydrate is under physiological control. Rats dramatically decrease their food intake when presented with a diet that is devoid of or has an excess of one essential amino acid. An amino acid deficiency appears to be monitored by the prepyriform cortex since electrolytic lesions of this area abolish the aversion of the rat to an amino acid imbalanced diet. Less is known about the control of amino acid excess, fat and carbohydrate selection. In contrast to the popular dictum that obese individuals "crave" carbohydrate, obese individuals prefer foods that are both high in fat and high in sugar. In the laboratory, genetically obese rats, when presented with individual sources of protein, fat and carbohydrate, also self-select diets high in fat. Adrenalectomy decreases fat selection and increases carbohydrate selection. Corticosterone replacement increases fat selection in a dose dependent fashion. While further research is needed to elucidate the precise mechanisms governing fat and carbohydrate selection, it is clear that palatability can play a major role.

REFERENCES

1. Blundell, J.E. (1983). Problems and processes underlying the control of food selection and nutrient intake. *In* "Nutrition and the Brain," Wurtman, R.J. and Wurtman, J.J., eds., Vol. 6, pp. 163-221. Raven Press, New York.
2. Castonguay, T.W., Applegate, E.A., Upton, D.E., and Stern, J.S. (1983). Hunger and appetite—old concepts/new distinctions. *Nutr. Rev.* **41**, 101-110.
3. Overmann, S.R. (1976). Dietary self-selection by animals. *Psychol. Bull.* **83**, 218-235.
4. Lat, J. (1967). Self selection of dietary components. *In* "Handbook of Physiology," Code, C.F., ed., Vol. 1, pp. 367-386. American Physiological Society, Washington, D.C.
5. Evvard, J.M. (1915). Is the appetite of swine a reliable indication of physiological needs? *Proc. Iowa Acad. Sci.* **22**, 375-403.
6. Osborne, T.B. and Mendel, L.B. (1918). The choice between adequate and inadequate diets as made by rats. *J. Biol. Chem.* **35**, 19-27.
7. Davis, C.M. (1928). Self selection of diet by newly weaned infants. *Am. J. Dis. Child.* **36**, 651-679.
8. Richter, C. (1939). Salt taste thresholds of normal and adrenalectomized rats. *Endocrinology* **24**, 367-371.
9. Richter, C. and Schmidt, E.C.H. (1939). Behavioral and anatomical changes produced in the rat by pancreatectomy. *Endocrinology* **21**, 50-54.
10. Gietzen, D.W., Leung, P.M.B., Castonguay, T.W., Hartman, W.J., and Rogers, Q.R. (1986). Time course of food intake and plasma and brain amino acid concentrations in rats fed amino acid-imbalanced or -deficient diets. *In* "Interaction of the Chemical Senses with Nutrition," Brand, J.G. and Kare, M.R., eds., pp. 415-456. Academic Press, New York, London.
11. Ashley, D.V.M. and Anderson, G.H. (1975). Correlation between the plasma tryptophan to neutral amino acid ratio and protein intake in the self-selecting weanling rat. *J. Nutr.* **105**, 1412-1421.
12. Peters, J.C. and Harper, A.E. (1981). Protein and energy consumption, plasma amino acid ratios, and brain neurotransmitter concentrations. *Physiol. Behav.* **27**, 287-298.
13. Leibowitz, S.F. (1986). Brain monoamines and peptides: role in the control of eating behavior. *Fed. Proc.* **45**, 1396-1403.
14. Leung, P.M-B. and Rogers, Q.R. (1971). Importance of pyriform cortex in food-intake response of rats to amino acids. *Am. J. Physiol.* **221**, 929-935.

15. Kanarek, R.B., Marks-Kaufman, R., and Lipeles, B.J. (1980). Increased carbohydrate intake as a function of insulin administration in rats. *Physiol. Behav.* **25**, 779-782.
16. Bellush, L.L. and Rowland, N. (1985). Preference for high carbohydrate over various high fat diets by diabetic rats. *Physiol. Behav.* **35**, 319-327.
17. Wurtman, J., Wurtman, R., Mack, S., Toay, R., Gilbert, W., and Growdon, J. (1985). d-Fenfluramine selectivity suppresses carbohydrate snacking by obese subjects. *Int. J. Eat. Disord.* **4**, 89-99.
18. Drewnowski, A. This volume, pp. 101-112.
19. Suzuki, M. and Tamura, T. This volume, pp. 113-119.
20. Castonguay, T.W., Hartman, W.J., Fitzpatrick, E.A., and Stern, J.S. (1982). Dietary self-selection and the Zucker rat. *J. Nutr.* **112**, 796-800.
21. Castonguay, T.W., Dallman, M.F., and Stern, J.S. (1986). Some metabolic and behavioral effects of adrenalectomy on obese Zucker rats. *Am. J. Physiol.* **251**, R923-933.
22. Grogan, C.K., Kim, H.-H., and Romsos, D.R. (1987). Effects of adrenalectomy on energy balance in obese (ob/ob) mice fed high carbohydrate or high fat diets. *J. Nutr.* **117**, 1115-1120.
23. Castonguay, T.W., Burdick, L., Guzman, M.A., Collier, G.H., and Stern, J.S. (1984). Self selection and the obese Zucker rat: the effect of dietary dilution. *Physiol. Behav.* **33**, 119-126.
24. Castonguay, T.W. and Stern, J.S. (1983). The effect of adrenalectomy on dietary component selection in obese and lean Zucker rats. *Nutr. Rep. Int.* **28**, 725-730.
25. Castonguay, T.W., Hirsch, E., and Collier, G.H. (1981). Palatability of sugar solutions and dietary selection. *Physiol. Behav.* **27**, 7-12.

Diet and Obesity, Bray, G.A. et al., eds., pp. 61-69.
Japan Sci. Soc. Press, Tokyo/S. Karger, Basel (1988)

Nervous and Endocrine Control of Meal Thermogenesis

JACQUES LeBLANC

Department of Physiology, School of Medicine, Laval University, Quebec P.Q., G1K 7P4, Canada

The maintenance of body temperature at around 37°C is made possible by the transformation of a high percentage of the energy intake into heat. In a sedentary lifestyle about 75% of the energy expenditure is due to resting metabolic rate (RMR), while 10 to 15% is used in physical activities and 10% by the processes involved in the digestion, absorption and storage of energy (*1*). This latter portion has been termed the thermic effect of feeding (TEF). The TEF, in the minds of many, has been essentially considered as synonymous with the specific dynamic action (SDA) of food as described by Rubner many years ago (*2*). It has been shown that the TEF varies according to the composition of the diet and to whether the nutrients are stored as lipids, proteins or glycogen (*3*). More recent studies, which are the object of the present review, indicate that the sensory stimulations associated with feeding may also have a direct action on TEF.

I. STUDIES ON HUMANS

In 1978 Rothwell and Stock published an article in Nature entitled "A paradox in the control of energy intake in the rat" (*4*). They fed one group of rats standard laboratory chow *ad libitum* and another group was given by stomach tube the same amount of calories. After 30 days the group fed by gavage had gained significantly more weight than the control group (Fig. 1). We proposed as a possible explanation for this unexpected finding that when the sensory stimulations normally associated with feeding (smell, taste and sight of food) are bypassed, the TEF is possibly reduced. To test this hypothesis a series of experiments was made on humans, dogs, and rats. In a first experiment, the TEF was measured when subjects ate a standard palatable meal and also when nutrients of the same composition and containing the same amount of calories were forced into the stomach through a nasal tube (*5*). It was found that normal feeding produced a significantly larger increase in TEF than tube feeding (Fig. 2). In another experiment, a palatable meal produced a more thermogenic response than when all the ingredients of the meal were blended together and presented to subjects as

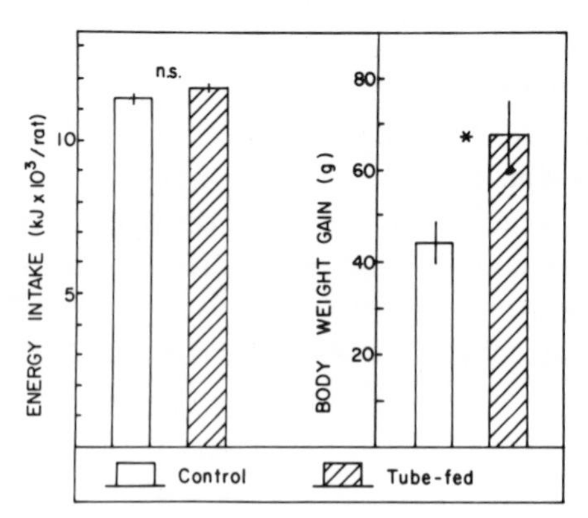

Fig. 1. Body weight gain of rats tube-fed for 30 days with energy intake similar to rats fed normally (*4*).

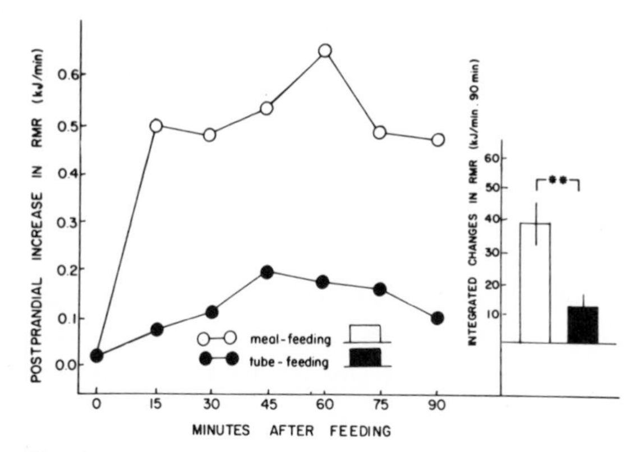

Fig. 2. Increase in RMR of subjects fed nutrients as a meal or by gastric tube (*5*).

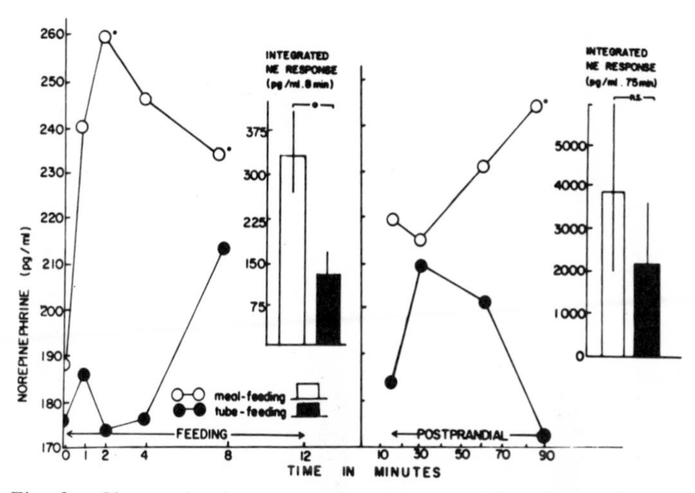

Fig. 3. Changes in plasma norepinephrine in subjects fed nutrients as a meal or by gastric tube (*6*).

a desiccated biscuit (*6*). In both these experiments feeding the palatable meal produced a significant elevation of plasma norepinephrine but tube-feeding and unpalatable food had no such effect (Fig. 3). Similarly, only the palatable food was found to increase the rapid so-called cephalic phase of insulin secretion. The findings in humans suggest the possible participation of the sympathetic nervous system in some component of TEF which could be independent of the SDA of food.

II. STUDIES ON DOGS

In order to elucidate the mechanism of this action, a series of experiments was done on dogs. This animal is a very gluttonous animal and it proved to be an excellent model for studies on TEF.

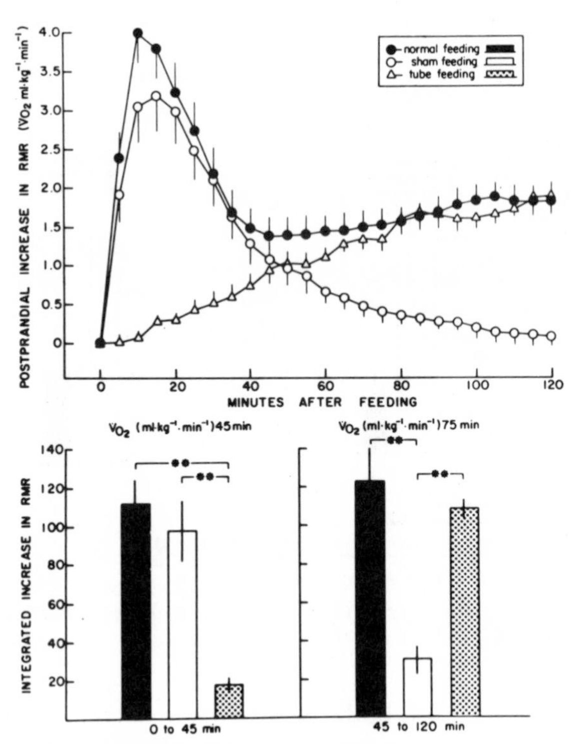

Fig. 4. Increase of RMR in dogs fed a standard meal, or when food is placed directly into the stomach (tube feeding) or collected into an oesophageal pouch after being swallowed (sham feeding) (7).

When fed a palatable meat-flavor meal, a rapid oxygen consumption increase is observed with value 100% above RMR within 15 min (Fig. 4). Sham feeding or the mere sight and smell of food caused as large an increase and it was found in this case that the increase above RMR lasted about 40 min (*7*). Thus, without any food ingestion, a 30% increase in thermogenesis was observed. During this cephalic phase marked increases in plasma insulin, norepinephrine and epinephrine were also observed (*8, 9*). With the injection of atropine or following vagal denervation of the pancreas, no rapid initial increase in plasma insulin was observed and a 40% reduction of TEF was noted. Pre-injection of a beta-blocker caused a similar reduction of TEF during the cephalic phase. When food was placed directly into the stomach through an oesophageal opening, the initial increase in TEF did not occur and the subsequent elevation in oxygen consumption, corresponding to the gastrointestinal phase of feeding was similar to that which results from normal feeding. As would be expected, this phase of TEF is blocked by atropine and is not observed with sham feeding. Thus the sympathetic and vagal components of the autonomic neurons are important in controlling TEF during the cephalic phase inasmuch as they stimulate norepinephrine and insulin secretion (*10*).

Studies have shown that obese people tend to eat fewer but larger meals than lean people (*11*). In order to test the thermogenic response to meal size and frequency, dogs were fed either a large meal representing the caloric requirements for 24 hr, or an equivalent intake in the form of four small meals fed at 1.5 hr intervals (*12*). The thermogenic response to the large meal was greater than that of the small meal during the gastrointestinal phase, but it was the same for both meal sizes during the cephalic phase (Fig. 5). It was also found that the total increase in postprandial oxygen consumption was about 100% higher when four small meals were fed instead of an isocaloric large meal. This result is not due to a difference in the gastrointestinal phase but solely to the fact that four cephalic phases were induced when the animals were fed the small meals instead of only once with the large meal.

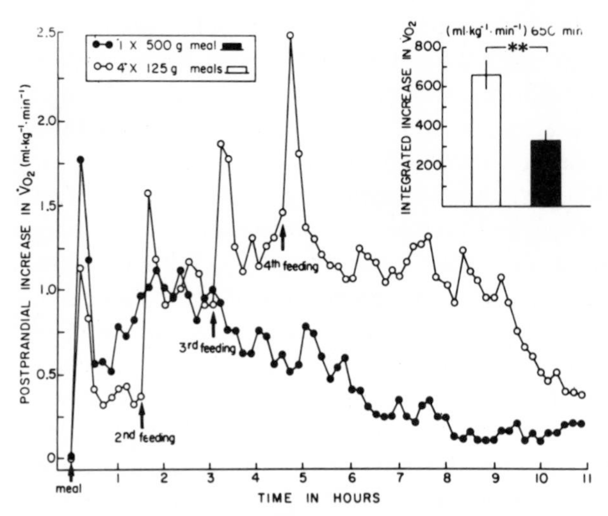

Fig. 5. Increase in RMR following one large meal (500 g) or 4 small meals (125 g) fed at 1.5 hr intervals (*12*).

III. STUDIES ON RATS

These acute experiments on men and on dogs suggest that the palatability of food may have a role to play in the control of body weight. This is not easy to prove with experiments on human subjects, but can be approached with studies done recently on rats (*13, 14*). Complete energy balance was made on three groups of rats fed for one month a control diet composed of standard laboratory pellets, a diet containing 50% of the control diet and 50% of a meat spread preparation, and the third group, a diet containing 50% of the control diet and 50% sugar pie fillings. Although the three groups were fed isocaloric diets, it was found that the body weight gain was smaller in the two groups fed the palatable meat spread or sugar pie fillings (Fig. 6). Carcass analysis showed that the energy expenditure was significantly larger in these two experimental groups. The enhanced response to norepinephrine and the elevation of protein concentration in the brown adipose tissue (BAT) in the groups fed palatable food suggest that the diet-induced thermogenesis (DIT)

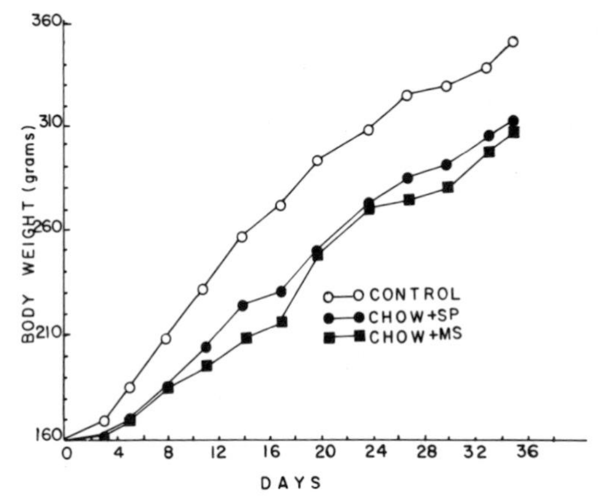

Fig. 6. Bodyweight changes in a control and two experimental pair-fed groups: CHOW refers to standard laboratory food, MS to meat spread, and SP to sugar pie fillings (*14*).

observed in these two groups is possibly related to an enhanced activity of the BAT. These results also indicate that excess food intake is not essential for producing DIT and that the composition of the diet is not an important factor, since meat spread with a high fat content and the sugar pie filling with its high carbohydrate concentration were equally efficient in increasing this regulatory thermogenesis. It is suggested from these studies on rats that palatability of food may play a significant role in DIT and in the control of body weight. The acute experiments on humans and on dogs have also shown that TEF can be produced by palatability of food (Fig. 7). It would be interesting to replicate on other species the experiments which were done on rats, especially in animals in which the thermogenic activity of BAT has not been unequivocally demonstrated.

SUMMARY

The thermic effect of feeding (TEF) which is due to the digestion absorption and storage of food has been shown to vary with the

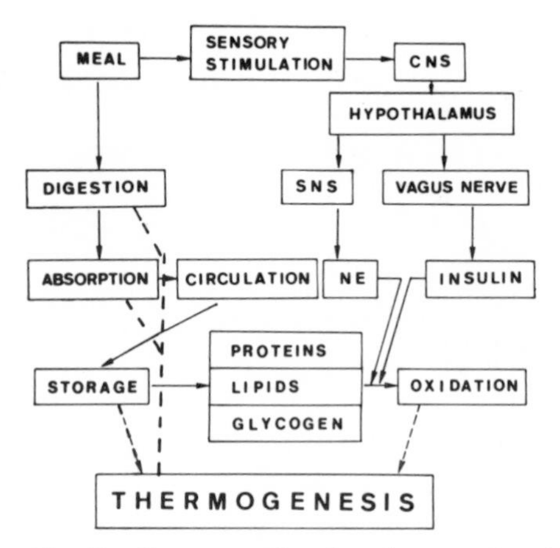

Fig. 7. Summary of various hormonal and nervous influences on meal thermogenesis. - - - sources of heat production; —— various influences.

composition of the meal and with the site of energy deposition. Recent studies indicate that sensory stimulations experienced during feeding also have a direct action on TEF. Results on humans have shown that unpalatable food or meal fed by gavage with a gastric tube were less thermogenic than eating an appetizing meal. Plasma norepinephrine was found to increase but only when the subjects ate a meal which they liked. These findings were confirmed on dogs. It was also shown in this species that an important part of thermogenesis observed during the cephalic phase of feeding is under both vagal and sympathetic influences. Long-term studies on rats suggest that the palatability of food may play a role in energy balance by increasing expenditure and reducing energy retention.

REFERENCES

1. Jéquier, E. (1981). Thermogenic regulation in man. *In* "Obesity: Pathogenesis and Treatment," Enzi, G. *et al.*, eds., pp. 45-55. Academic Press, New York.
2. Rubner, M. (1902). Die Gesetze des Energievrebranchs bie der Ernahrung. Dauticke, Leipzig.
3. Flatt, J.P. (1977). The biochemistry of energy expenditure. *In* "Recent Advances

in Obesity Research II," Bray, G., ed., pp. 211-228. Newman, Washington, D.C.
4. Rothwell, N.J. and Stock, M.J. (1978). A paradox in the control of energy intake in the rat. *Nature* **273**, 146-147.
5. LeBlanc, J., Cabanac, M., and Samson, P. (1984). Reduced postprandial heat production with gavage as compared with meal feeding in human subjects. *Am. J. Physiol.* **246**, E95-E101.
6. LeBlanc, J. and Brondel, L. (1985). Role of palatability on meal induced thermogenesis in human subjects. *Am. J. Physiol.* **248**, E333-E336.
7. Diamond, P., Brondel, L., and LeBlanc, J. (1985). Palatability and postprandial thermogenesis in dogs. *Am. J. Physiol.* **248**, E75-E79.
8. Diamond, P. and LeBlanc, J. (1987). Hormonal control of postprandial thermogenesis in dogs. *Am. J. Physiol.* **252**, E719-726.
9. Diamond, P. and LeBlanc, J. (1987). A role for insulin in the cephalic phase of postprandial thermogenesis in dogs. *Am. J. Physiol.* **254**, E625-632.
10. Diamond, P. and LeBlanc, J. (1987). Role of the autonomic nervous system in postprandial thermogenesis in dogs. *Am. J. Physiol.* **252**, E719-E726.
11. Adams, C.E. and Morgan, K.J. (1981). Periodicity of eating: implications for human food consumption. *Nutr. Res.* **11**, 525-550.
12. LeBlanc, J. and Diamond, P. (1986). Effect of meal size and frequency on postprandial thermogenesis. *Am. J. Physiol.* **250**, E144-E147.
13. Allard, M. and LeBlanc, J. (1987). Effect of cold acclimation, cold exposure and palatability of diet on postprandial thermogenesis in rats. *Int. J. Obesity* **12**, 169-176.
14. LeBlanc, J. and Allard, M. (1987). Body weight reduction produced by isocaloric palatable food. *Can. J. Physiol. Pharmacol.*, submitted.

Diet and Obesity, Bray, G.A. et al., eds., pp. 71–85.
Japan Sci. Soc. Press, Tokyo/S. Karger, Basel (1988)

Regulation of Diet-induced Thermogenesis in Brown Adipose Tissue

LUDWIK J. BUKOWIECKI

Department of Physiology, Laval University Medical School, Quebec, P.Q. G1K 7P4, Canada

It has been known for approximately 25 years that brown adipose tissue (BAT) represents an important site of cold-induced thermogenesis (nonshivering thermogenesis) in homeotherms (*1–3*). Ten years ago several research groups postulated that thermogenesis can be stimulated in BAT, not only by cold exposure, but also by overfeeding palatable diets (diet-induced thermogenesis (DIT) (*4–6*). Cold exposure and overfeeding palatable diets both stimulate the activity of the sympathetic nervous system (SNS), albeit *via* different mechanisms that remain to be elucidated (*7, 8*). This results in a release of noradrenaline from nerve fibers surrounding individual brown adipocytes (*9*). Noradrenaline activates thermogenesis in brown adipocytes by stimulating lipolysis and respiration mainly *via* beta-1 adrenergic receptors (in the rat) (*10*), but the role of other receptors (alpha 1-2, beta-2 or "atypical" beta) still remains to be evaluated, particularly in species other than the rat (*8*) (Fig. 1).

The physiological function of DIT is to burn the excess of calories ingested after overfeeding palatable diets in order to prevent

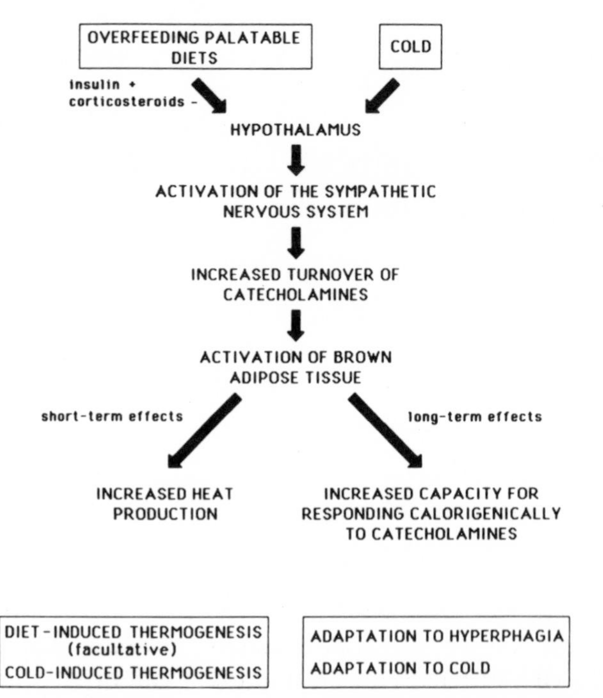

Fig. 1. Stimulation of BAT thermogenesis by cold exposure and by overfeeding palatable diets *via* activation of the SNS. The diagram also shows that animals can adapt to cold and/or to hyperphagia by increasing their capacity for responding calorigenically to catecholamines. Insulin and glucocorticoids modulate the activity of the SNS.

excessive weight gain. Thus, a defective activation of DIT in BAT should theoretically lead to an increased energy gain efficiency that would result, at long-term, in obesity. It is remarkable that a defective DIT in BAT has been identified in several different models of animal obesity: the *ob/ob* mouse, the *fa/fa* Zucker rat, the ventromedial hypothalamic-lesioned rat and the gold-thioglucose treated mouse (for reviews, *4–6*). The mechanisms leading to a defective thermogenesis in these four models of animal obesity are likely to be different. *A priori*, the defect might reside at the level of stimulus recognition (diet) by the hypothalamus or in the control of the SNS by insulin, glucocorticoids, *etc.*. A defect might also be present in BAT itself, for instance, at the level of the mitochondrial uncoupling protein. However, it is more likely that the defect explaining the increased energy gain efficiency of animal models of obesity is multifactorial and might involve complex interactions between diet composition and neuroendocrine regulation (*11*). Nevertheless, the fact remains that obesity can be achieved without hyperphagia in all the above animal models (as demonstrated by pair-feeding experiments) and that BAT represents one of the anatomical sites of the decreased thermogenesis.

On the other hand, it is known that rats and other small mammals possess the ability of adapting to cold as well as to hyperphagia by increasing their capacity for responding calorigenically to catecholamines. This phenomenon is characterized by a remarkable hyperplasia of brown adipose tissue that represents the physiological explanation for the hyperadrenergic response of cold-acclimated and/or hyperphagic animals to catecholamines (*1-6, 13-15*). Thus, the capacity of the animals for DIT may be increased by long-term overfeeding with palatable diets.

In this communication, we shall first analyze the hormonal mechanisms controlling BAT thermogenesis and next the physiological and pharmacological mechanisms regulating the capacity of brown adipose tissue for cold- and diet-induced thermogenesis.

I. HORMONAL REGULATION OF BAT THERMOGENESIS

Nordrenaline is the principal, but not the sole effector of thermogenesis in BAT. The fundamental role of noradrenaline can easily be demonstrated by denervating interscapular BAT. This results in an increased BAT lipid content, a decreased BAT growth in the cold and a decreased thermogenic capacity (see ref. *8*). Noradrenaline activates thermogenesis in isolated brown adipocytes by stimulating lipolysis (*10, 15, 16*). Fatty acids (or their acyl CoA derivatives), released in consequence of stimulated lipolysis, elicit thermogenesis by increasing mitochondrial permeability to protons at the level of the uncoupling protein (*17, 18*). Long-chain fatty

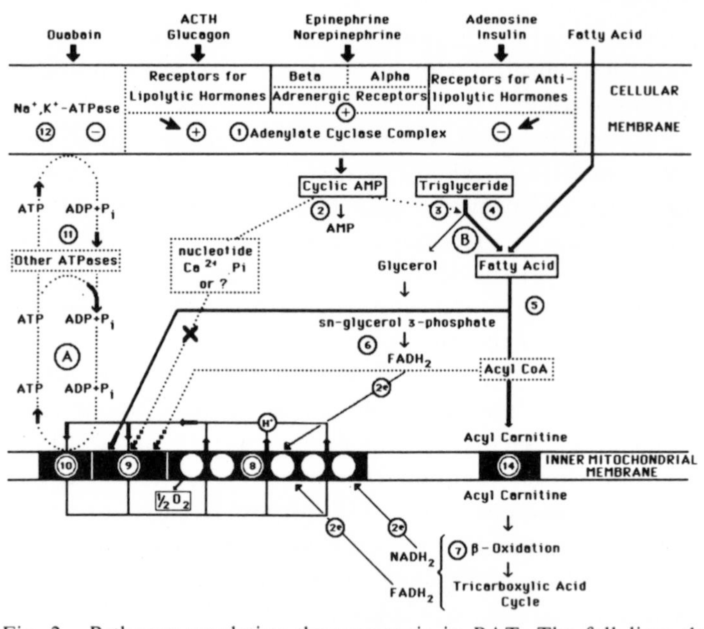

Fig. 2. Pathways regulating thermogenesis in BAT. The full lines denote well-established pathways, whereas the broken lines represent hypothetical pathways regulating thermogenesis. Pathways of lipolysis and oxidative phosphorylation are shown in outline: (1) the hormone-sensitive adenylate cyclase complex localized in the cell membrane in association with hormonal receptors, (2) cAMP phosphodiesterase, (3) the system of protein kinases, (4) triglyceride lipases, (5) fatty acid activating enzymes, (6) glycerophosphate dehydrogenase, (7) metabolic systems generating reduced coenzymes, (8) the electron transport chain and the pumping of protons across the inner mitochondrial membrane generating an electrochemical gradient, (9) mitochondrial proton conductance pathways (uncoupling protein) controlling proton re-entry into the matrix responsible for the dissipation of the proton electrochemical gradient, (10) oligomycin-sensitive ATP synthetase driven by the proton electrochemical gradient, (11) Ca^{2+}-ATPases and other ATPases, (12) (Na^{+}-K^{+})-ATPase localized in the plasma membrane. The sign X indicates an unlikely metabolic pathway because it has been demostrated that fatty acids stimulate respiration when cAMP production is inhibited by propranolol. This sign refers to a hypothetical sequence of metabolic events triggered by norepinephrine and does not indicate that nucleotides or other ions are unnecessary for the control of mitochondrial respiration. (A) represents respiration controlled by cellular ATPases. (B) represents respiration controlled by lipolysis.

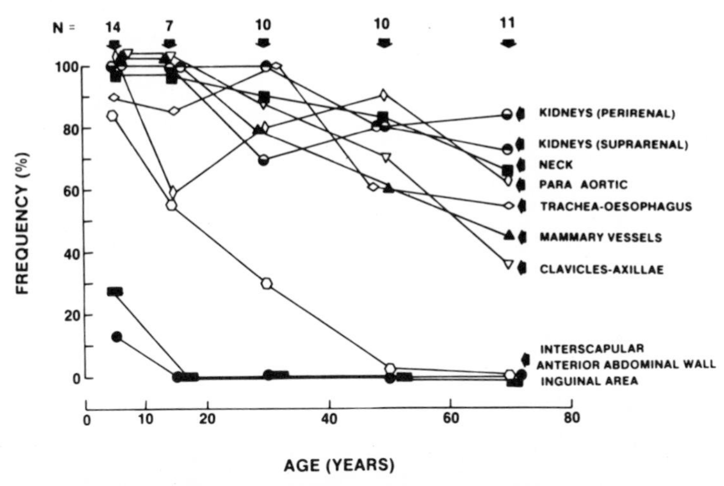

Fig. 3. The distribution of BAT in the human. The graph represents the frequency of finding typical brown adipocytes (identified by light microscopy) in various adipose depots in infants and adult humans who had died suddenly. N denotes the number of subjects for each age group (52 subjects). It can be seen that BAT was found in nearly all adipose tissue depots obtained from 0–10 year old children. With age, BAT gradually disappeared in certain adipose depots while it remained present in others, particularly around the kidneys. The probability of finding BAT around the kidneys was approximately 80% for 60–80 year old people. Adapted from J.M. Heaton (1972). *J. Anat.* **112**, 35–39.

acids stimulate thermogenesis in isolated brown adipocytes even in the presence of propranolol, *i.e.*, when cAMP production is blocked (Fig. 2, section B). This demonstrates that increased cAMP production *per se* is not required for uncoupling oxidative phosphorylation and that fatty acids (or their acyl CoA derivatives) represent the "metabolic messengers" between lipolysis and respiration. The evidence that lipolysis and respiration are tightly coupled metabolic processes has recently been reviewed (*19*). However, it should be pointed out that the control of respiration by fatty acids is a self-regulatory process: fatty acids retro-inhibit lipolysis if added in excess to isolated brown adipocytes (*15*). Studies in which ouabain was used for blocking the Na-K ATPase demonstrated that nora-

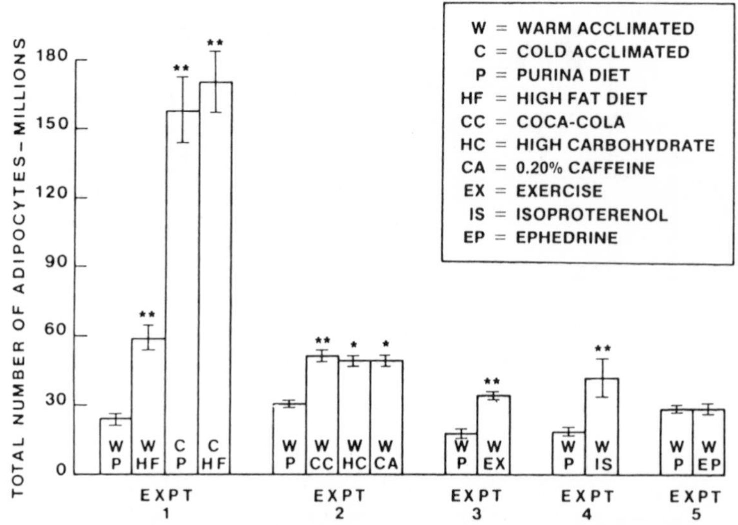

Fig. 4. Modulation of BAT cellularity. The figure summarizes results from five different experiments performed on separate occasions in which the effects of various treatments on the cellularity of interscapular BAT were evaluated. All experiments were performed with female Wistar rats weighing 175–200 g at the beginning of the treatments. Exp. 1 (for details see ref. *13*): the animals were in four groups: two groups were exposed to the cold (40°C) for 10 weeks (C) and two others were maintained in the warm (25°C) for the same period of time (W). One group in the warm and one group in the cold were allowed a "cafeteria" diet that represented mainly a high fat diet (HF), whereas the other groups were given Purina chow (P). Exp. 2 (for details see ref. *14*): the animals were also divided into four groups but they were all maintained at 25°C and had free access to Purina chow. The control group was maintained as usual on tap water. However, the first experimental group was given Coca-Cola *ad libitum* instead of water, another group was given sucrose at approximately the same concentration as in Coca-Cola whereas the the third experimental group was given 0.20% ca1eine dissolved in tap water. Exp. 3: the experimental animals were submitted to an endurance exercise training program that consisted of 2–3 hr of daily swimming over a period of 6–10 weeks. The temperature of the water was maintained at 35–36°C to avoid a cold stress. Exp. 4: the experimental animals received subcutaneous injections of the beta adrenergic agonist isoproterenol (700 μg/kg), twice a day, during a period of 4 weeks. Control animals were similarly injected with the carrier solution. Exp. 5: the experimental animals received daily doses (p.o.) of ephedrine (50 mg/kg) during a period of 9–10 weeks. It might be pointed out that animals on caffeine (*13*) and ephedrine significantly lost body weight.

drenaline might also activate thermogenesis by stimulating the NA-K-ATPase, but this pathway represents only 15% of the total calorigenic effects of the neurohormone (Fig. 2, section A).

In addition to noradrenaline and fatty acids, brown adipocyte thermogenesis can be stimulated *in vitro* by a variety of lipolytic hormones (adrenaline, glucagon, adrenocorticotropic hormone, thyroid-stimulating hormone) or lipolytic drugs (caffeine, theophylline, 3-isobutyl-1-methylxanthine, dcAMP, ephedrine, adrenergic agonists, *etc.*). Likewise, noradrenaline-stimulated thermogenesis is inhibited by anti-lipolytic agents (insulin, prostaglandins, adenosine, adrenergic antagonists, *etc.*) (*19*). Insulin does not stimulate BAT thermogenesis *in vitro* (*19*) or *in vivo* in anesthetized animals (in which the activity of the SNS is depressed) (*20*). It is therefore likely that insulin stimulates BAT thermogenesis indirectly, by activating the SNS (*7*).

II. REGULATION OF BAT CELLULARITY

Brown adipose tissue has the ability to grow and regress according to the need for thermogenesis. It is particularly abundant in newborn mammals, including man (*21–23*). If the newborn animals are not exposed to cold, brown adipocytes progressively de-differentiate into cells resembling white adipocytes (Fig. 3). Indeed, during animal growth the body surface/volume ratio decreases and the need for a tissue specialized in heat production diminishes. In addition, many mammals develop a layer of insulating fat under an abundant fur. Man protects himself against cold with warm clothes.

Nevertheless, cells capable of differentiating into brown adipocytes remain present in adult animals, even in adult men. If these cells (interstitial cells) are stimulated by cold exposure, hyperphagia (either high fat or high carbohydrate diets), catecholamine infusions (norepinephrine or isoproterenol) or epinephrine (phaeochromocytoma), they rapidly differentiate into brown adipocytes (*17, 23–25*) (Fig. 4). Using tritiated thymidine to follow mitoses by autoradiography, we recently demonstrated that the stimulation of BAT

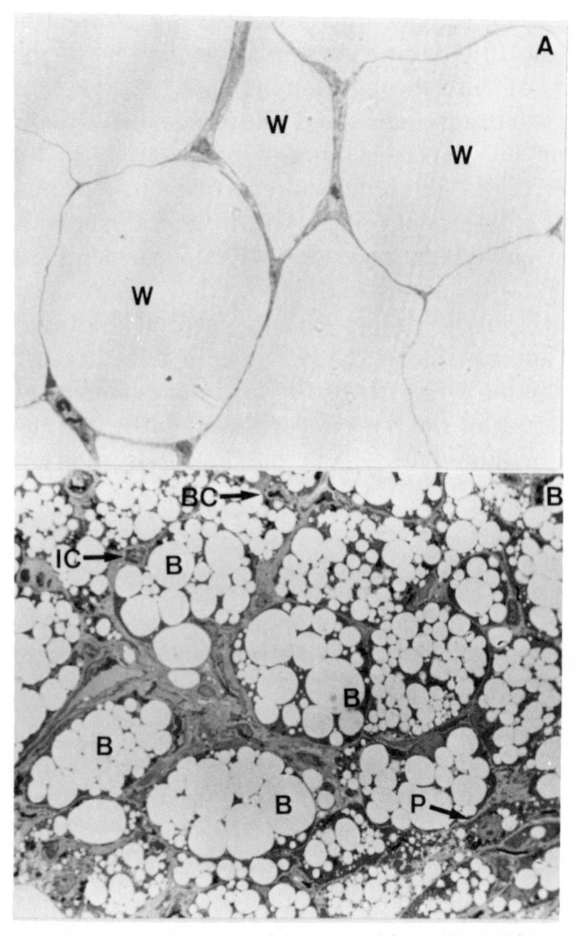

Fig. 5. General aspect of human white adipose tissue and BAT by light microscopy (1 μ sections). The patient was a 64 year old woman who had a nephrectomy. A: white adipose tissue from the abdominal region. All adipocytes (W) are unilocular. Magnification: $\times$1,700. B: BAT from the perirenal region. Magnification: $\times$1,700. Typical brown adipocytes (B) are smaller cells (diameter of 15-25 μm) than white adipocytes (W). A small brown preadipocyte (P) in which a nucleus and two nucleoli can be seen is tentatively identified. Interstitial cells (IC) are very small cells that do not contain triglyceride droplets and which probably represent the precursors of pre brown adipocytes. BC, blood capillaries.

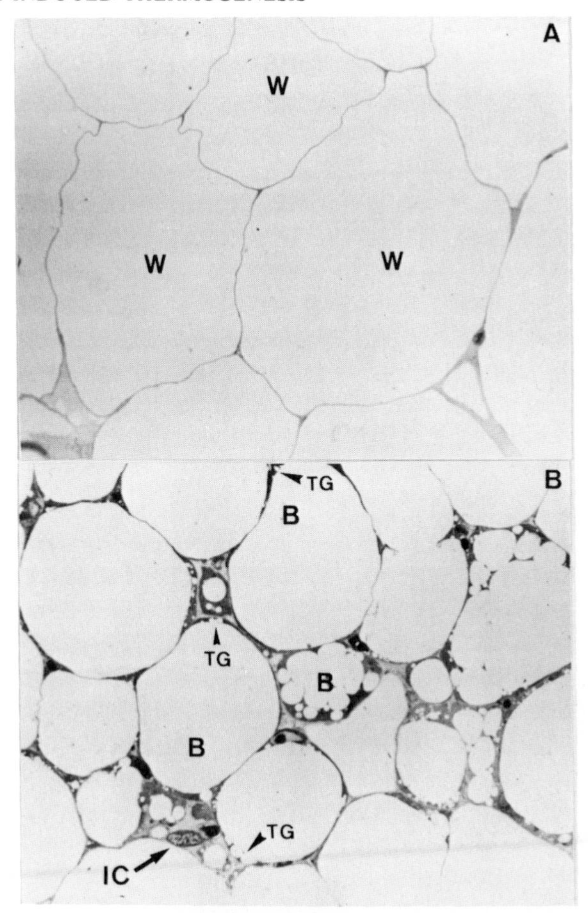

Fig. 6. General aspect of human white adipose tissue and BAT by light microscopy (1 μm sections). The patient was a 59 year old woman who had a nephrectomy. A: white adipose tissue from the abdominal region. All adipocytes (W) are unilocular. Magnification: $\times$1,700. B: BAT from the perirenal region. Magnification: $\times$1,700. Note that some of the small brown adipocytes (B) are multilocular whereas other brown adipocytes are apparently unilocular. In fact, a closer examination of their cytoplasm reveals the presence of tiny triglyceride droplets (TG). An interstitial cell (IC) with an elongated dense nucleus does not contain triglyceride droplets. BC, blood capillaries.

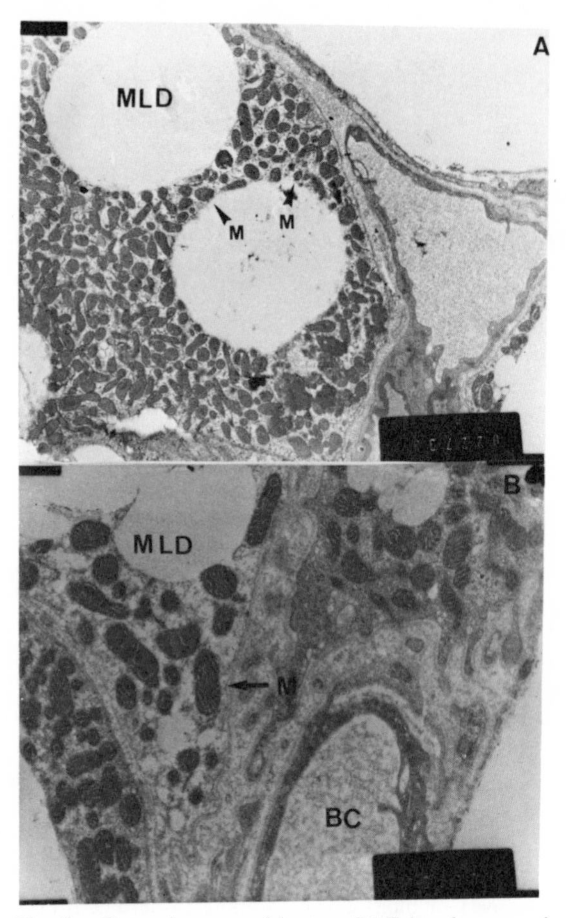

Fig. 7. General aspect of human BAT by electron microscopy. The patient was the same as in Fig. 5. Magnification: A, ×7,000; B, ×17,000. MLD, multilocular lipid droplets. Note the numerous mitochondria (M) with tightly packed cristae seen in their condensed (thermogenic ?) conformation. BC, blood capillary.

proliferative activity by cold exposure could be mimicked by infusing norepinephrine or isoproterenol in warm-exposed animals. The alpha adrenergic agonist phenylephrine was unable to stimulate mitoses in BAT (*25*).

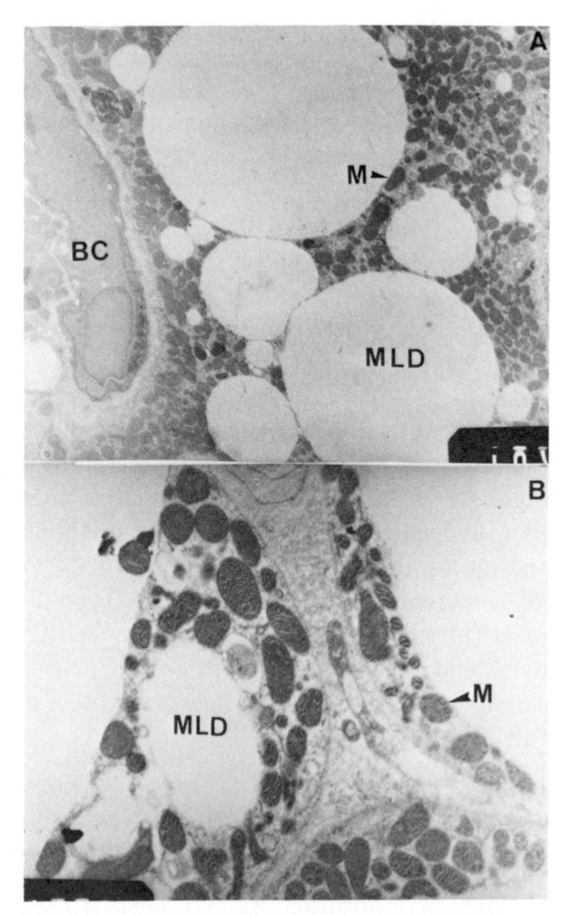

Fig. 8. General aspect of human brown adipose tissue by electron microscopy. The patient was same as in Fig. 6. Magnification: A, ×7,000; B, ×17,000. MLD, multilocular lipid droplets. Note the tightly packed cristae seen in their condensed (thermogenic ?) conformation. BC, blood capillary.

III. BAT IN HUMANS

Brown adipose tissue has been identified in adult humans by biochemical (uncoupling protein concentration) and ultrastructural methods (see *17, 22, 26*) (Figs. 5-8). The evidence that BAT is functional in humans is indirect. Man responds calorigenically to catecholamines, caffeine, and ephedrine as animals do, but the magnitude of the response is much smaller. The fact that old fat rats, adult pigs and genetically obese animals do not respond well to catecholamines or possess a reduced sympathetic activity suggests that certain forms of obesity might be explained by a thermogenic defect in DIT, but this still remains to be directly demonstrated. Thus, there is no reason to believe at the present time that the thermogenic responses to a meal are qualitatively different in man and laboratory animals. Hyperphagia is certainly the main cause of human obesity, but it is not the cause of what has been called "refractory obesity". Obesity without hyperphagia may occur in man as it does in laboratory animals. It would therefore appear interesting to differentiate *metabolic* from *hyperphagic* obesity in clinical studies. The calorigenic response to caffeine might serve as a simple tool for testing the thermogenic capacity of obese people. This might lead to a classification of obesity in Type I (high responders) or Type II (low responders). Attempts to classify obese people as "high eaters" and "low eaters" might also be helpful. The time has come to classify obesity in various categories, as was done a long time ago with diabetes.

IV. CONCLUSION

There are at least four types of evidence indicating that BAT is a site of facultative DIT in laboratory animals:(1) a single meal activates thermogenesis in BAT, (2) prolonged hyperphagia (during weeks) increases BAT capacity for thermogenesis, (3) surgical removal of interscapular BAT leads to an increased energy gain efficiency that may result in obesity, and (4) several animal models of obesity (*ob/ob* mice, *fa/fa* Zucker rats, hypothalamic obesity, *etc.*) display a reduced thermogenesis in their BAT that may be consequent to a decreased sympathetic activity. Further research should concentrate on the quantitative contribution of BAT thermogenesis for total DIT.

SUMMARY

1. The hormonal and biochemical mechanisms regulating DIT in BAT will be briefly reviewed. The principal trigger of diet- and cold-induced thermogenesis in BAT is noradrenaline released from sympathetic nerves but other hormones (insulin, adenosine, glucagon, glucocorticoids) may modulate thermogenesis. Studies with isolated brown adipocytes revealed that long-chain fatty acids represent the metabolic messenger between lipolysis and respiration. In general, lipolytic agents (glucagon, adrenocorticotropic hormone, adrenergic drugs, methylxanthines, *etc.*) stimulate BAT respiration whereas thermogenic agents (insulin, adenosine, adrenergic antagonists) inhibit respiration. Thus, the hormone-sensitive lipases represent the flux-generating step regulating BAT respiration.

2. BAT posses the ability to grow when its thermogenic function is chronically stimulated by diet (hyperphagia), cold exposure or drugs. In the rat, BAT hyperplasia represents the physiological explanation for the hyperadrenergic response of cold-acclimated and/or hyperphagic animals. A defective DIT in BAT has been identified in several animal models of obesity (*ob/ob* mice, the Zucker rat, hypothalamic obesity). It is therefore possible that BAT plays the role of an energy buffering system and that a defective DIT leads to a higher energy gain efficiency that characterizes certain models of obesity.

3. BAT is present in humans, even in 60–80 years adults. Indirect evidence suggests that it is functional but the quantitative contribution of BAT to total energy expenditure is unknown. Although hyperphagia represents the main cause of obesity, a defective DIT in BAT may contribute to refractory obesity (obesity without hyperphagia). It would be helpful to classify human obesity in various categories (metabolic or hyperphagic obesity) and not to consider all obese people guilty of ferocious voracity.

REFERENCES

1. Smith, R.F. and Horwitz, B.A. (1969). Brown fat thermogenesis. *Physiol. Rev.* **49**, 330-425.
2. Jansky, L. (1973). Non-shivering thermogenesis and its thermoregulatory significance. *Biol. Rev.* **48**, 85-132.
3. Foster, D.O. (1986). Quantitative role of brown adipose tissue in thermogenesis, *In* "Brown Adipose Tissue," Trayhurn, P. and Nicholls, D., eds., pp. 31-51. Arnold A.E., London.
4. Trayhurn, P. (1986). Brown adipose tissue and energy balance. *In* "Brown Adipose Tissue," Trayhurn, P. and Nicholls, D., eds., pp. 299-338. Arnold A.E., London.
5. Rothwell, N.J. and Stock, M.J. (1986). Brown adipose tissue and diet-induced thermogenesis. *In* "Brown Adipose Tissue," Trayhurn, P. and Nicholls, D., eds., pp. 269-238. Arnold A.E., London.
6. Himms-Hagen, J. (1986). Brown adipose tissue and cold-acclimation. *In* "Brown Adipose Tissue," Trayhurn, P. and Nicholls, D., eds., pp. 214-268. Arnold A.E., London.
7. Landsberg, L. and Young, J.B. (1983). Autonomic regulation of thermogenesis. *In* "Mammalian Thermogenesis," Girardier, L. and Stock, M.J., eds., pp. 99-140. Chapman and Hall, London.
8. Girardier, L. and Seydoux, J. (1986). Neural control of brown adipose tissue. *In* "Brown Adipose Tissue," Trayhurn, P. and Nicholls, D., eds., pp. 122-151. Arnold A.E., London.
9. Cottle, M.K.V., Cottle, W. H., Perusse, F., and Bukowiecki, L. J. (1985). An improved glyoxylic acid technique for the histochemical localization of catecholamines in brown adipose tissue. *Histochem. J.* **17**, 1279-1288.
10. Bukowiecki, L., Follea, N., Paradis, A., and Collet, A.J. (1980). Stereospecific stimulation of brown adipose tissue respiration by catecholamines via beta 1-adrenergic receptors. *Am. J. Physiol.* **238**, E552-E563.
11. Kim, H.-K. and Romsos, D. (1987). Brown adipose tissue thermogenesis in *ob/ob* mice: effects of a high-fat diet and adrenalectomy. *Am. J. Physiol.* **253**, E149-E157.
12. Jansky, L. (1973). Non-shivering thermogenesis and its thermoregulatory significance. *Biol. Rev.* **48**, 85-132.
13. Bukowiecki, L., Collet, A.J., Follea, N., Guay, G., and Jahjah, L. (1982). Brown adipose tissue hyperplasia: a fundamental mechanism of adaptation to cold and hyperphagia. *Am. J. Physiol.* **242**, E353-E359.
14. Bukowiecki, L., Lupien, J., Follea, N., and Jahjah, L. (1983). Effects of sucrose, caffeine and cola beverages on the resistance of rats to cold and on the cellularity of brown and white adipose tissues. *Am. J. Physiol.* **244**, R500-R507.

15. Bukowiecki, L., Follea, N., Lupien, J., and Paradis, A. (1981). Metabolic interrelationships between lipolysis and respiration in rat brown adipocytes. The role of long-chain fatty acids as regulators of mitochondrial respiration and feedback inhibitors of lipolysis. *J. Biol. Chem.* **256**, 12840-12848.
16. Szillat, D. and Bukowiecki, L. (1983). Control of brown adipose tissue respiration by adenosine. *Am. J. Physiol.* **245**, E555-E559.
17. Ricquier, D. and Bouillaud, F. (1986). The brown adipose tissue mitochondrial uncoupling protein. *In* "Brown Adipose Tissue," Trayhurn, P. and Nicholls, D., eds., pp. 86-104. Arnold A.E., London.
18. Nicholls, D.G., Cunningham, S., and Rial, E. (1986). The bioenergetic mechanisms of brown adipose tissue mitochondria. *In* "Brown Adipose Tissue," Trayhurn, P. and Nicholls, D., eds., pp 52-85. Arnold A.E., London.
19. Bukowiecki, L. (1986). Lipid metabolism in brown adipose tissue. *In* "Brown Adipose Tissue," Trayhurn, P. and Nicholls, D., eds., pp. 105-121. Arnold A.E., London.
20. Shibata, H., Perusse, F., and Bukowiecki, L.J. (1986). The role of insulin in nonshivering thermogenesis. *Can. J. Physiol. Pharmacol.* **65**, 152-158.
21. Nedergaard, J., Connolly, E., and Cannon, B. (1986). Brown adipose tissue in the mammalian neonate. *In* "Brown Adipose Tissue," Trayhurn, P. and Nicholls, D., eds., pp. 152-213. Arnold A.E., London.
22. Lean, M.E.J. and James, W.P.T. Brown adipose tissue in man. *In* "Brown Adipose Tissue," Trayhurn, P. and Nicholls, D., eds., pp. 339-366. Arnold A.E., London.
23. Nechad, M. (1986). Structure and development of brown adipose tissue. *In* "Brown Adipose Tissue," Trayhurn, P. and Nicholls, D., eds., pp. 1-30. Arnold A.E., London.
24. Bukowiecki, L.J., Geloen, A., and Collet A.J. (1986). Proliferation and differentiation of brown adipocytes from interstitial cells during cold acclimation. *Am. J. Physiol.* **250**, C880-887.
25. Geloen, A., Collet, A.J., Guay, and Bukowiecki, L.J. (1987). Beta-adrenergic stimulation of brown adipocyte proliferation. *Am. J. Physiol.* **254**, C175-182.
26. Bukowiecki, L. and Collet, A.J. (1983). Regulation of brown adipose tissue metabolism. *J. Obesity Weight Regul.* **2**, 29-53.

Diet and Obesity, Bray, G.A. et al., eds., pp. 87-100.
Japan Sci. Soc. Press, Tokyo/S. Karger, Basel (1988)

Efficiency of Carbohydrate and Fat Utilization for Oxidation and Storage

JEAN-PIERRE FLATT

Department of Biochemistry, University of Massachusetts Medical School, Worcester, MA 01655, U.S.A.

When compared to daily energy turnover, the amount of energy retained during the development of obesity is quite small. A gain of 2 kg of adipose tissue fat over a one year period, which one would consider to be quite significant for an adult, amounts to an average gain of only 50 kcal/day. This represents a cumulative difference of but 2% between energy intake and expenditure. Such considerations have greatly contributed to elicit interest in the possible role of small differences in metabolic efficiency as a factor contributing to the development of obesity (*1*).

I. METABOLIC EFFICIENCY

Metabolic efficiency can be defined in various ways (Table I). Relating energy deposited in the carcass to total amount of food energy consumed has long been an important practical relationship to judge feed efficiency in the production of meat. The efficiency value yielded by this expression rises progressively with increasing amounts of excess energy consumed. But in a situation characterized

TABLE I
Possible Basis for Defining Metabolic Efficiency

$\frac{\text{Energy retained}}{\text{Energy intake}}$		$\frac{\text{Energy retained}}{\text{Energy intake above requirement}}$
$\frac{\text{Work produced}}{\text{Energy intake}}$		$\frac{\text{Work produced}}{\Delta\text{Metabolic rate}}$
$\frac{\Delta\text{Metabolic rate}}{\text{Amount of nutrients ingested}}$		$\frac{\Delta\text{Metabolic rate}}{\text{Amount of nutrients stored}}$
	$\frac{\text{Energy required for maintenance}}{\text{Normal energy requirement for maintenance}}$	
	$\frac{\text{Energy required for activities}}{\text{Normal energy requirement for activities}}$	
$\frac{\text{ATP made}}{\text{kcal expended}}$	$\frac{\text{ATP replaced}}{\text{ATP generated}}$	$\frac{\text{ATP replaced}}{\text{kcal expended}}$

by rather small changes in body size over time, such as in adult man, metabolic efficiencies calculated by this criterion would be close to zero. Dealing with metabolic efficiencies near 0% is hardly helpful in trying to understand metabolic features.

Expressing metabolic efficiency in terms of energy retained relative to energy consumed in excess of maintenance requirements may appear to be a more useful approach. It is difficult to apply this definition, however, because energy requirements for maintenance keep changing as body weight varies. Furthermore, one may wonder whether it is rational to extrapolate to total metabolic turnover an efficiency value based on consideration of the fate of calories consumed in excess.

A much more precise circumstance for measuring metabolic efficiency is offered by relating the amount of work produced to the change in metabolic rate which it causes. Typical values obtained in animals and man for aerobic exertion are in the vicinity of 27% (*2, 3*). These values are quite reproducible for a given type of exercise. The cost of weight bearing activities is roughly proportional to body weight (*4*). No difference in work efficiency between normal and obese subjects has been found (*5*).

II. THERMIC EFFECT OF FOODS

The "thermic effect of foods" (TEF) (formally called "specific dynamic action" of food) can be measured quite accurately as well, particularly in man who is a cooperating experimental subject. One half to two thirds of the TEF can usually be attributed to the ATP expenditure required to store the ingested nutrients. This "obligatory" component of the TEF (*6*) can be assessed more precisely when indirect calorimetry measurements are available, which allow calculation of the actual amounts of nutrients stored. Assuming that an increment in energy expenditure of 20 kcal is required to regenerate 1 mol of ATP consumed in the process of nutrient storage, the obligatory costs amount to about 7% of the carbohydrate effectively converted to glycogen (*7*), or usually to some 5% of carbohydrate energy consumed, since some of the glucose ingested is oxidized without prior storage. The TEF commonly observed for carbohydrate varies from 7 to 10%. This is because additional energy expenditure is elicited by stimulation of the sympathetic nervous system. This phenomenon is commonly referred to as the "facultative" component of TEF. It can be suppressed by propranolol, a beta-blocker, and the observed TEF then becomes similar to the predicted obligatory TEF (*6*). Carbohydrate, but not protein or fat, elicits this catecholamine-mediated increase in energy expenditure (*8*). The latter also appears to be enhanced by the palatability of the foods consumed (*9*), and it is greater after oral ingestion of a palatable meal than after delivery of the same foods by a stomach tube (*10*). A decrease in the thermic effect of food has been observed in some obese subjects following appreciable weight loss (*11*).

Much greater metabolic costs are incurred if ingested carbohydrate is converted into fat. The cost of fatty acid synthesis from glucose consumes an amount of energy equivalent to 20% of carbohydrate calories channeled into the lipogenic pathway (*7*), or some 25% if the costs for prior conversion to glycogen plus transport and deposition into adipose tissue are also considered. Non-protein respiratory quotients (RQ's) above 1.0 indicate that lipogenesis exceeds the concomitant rate of fat oxidation. High rates of lipogenesis can be induced in man by prolonged intake of massive excesses of carbohydrate calories, once accumulation of about 500 g of glycogen has occurred (*12*). After 7 days of consuming an excess of 1,500 kcal of carbohydrate per day the non-protein RQ was 1.15 and an increase in resting metabolic rate of 35% was observed. Three quarters of this increase was due to the obligatory component of the TEF (*12*). After ingestion of a single 500 g load of carbohydrate, the non-protein RQ will only transiently exceed 1.0 (Fig. 1), as a gain of 400 g of glycogen can be accommodated before this occurs (*13*). People consuming a mixed diet will not commonly consume such large amounts of carbohydrates, and conversion of carbohydrate into fat appears to be a minor metabolic process under generally prevailing conditions.

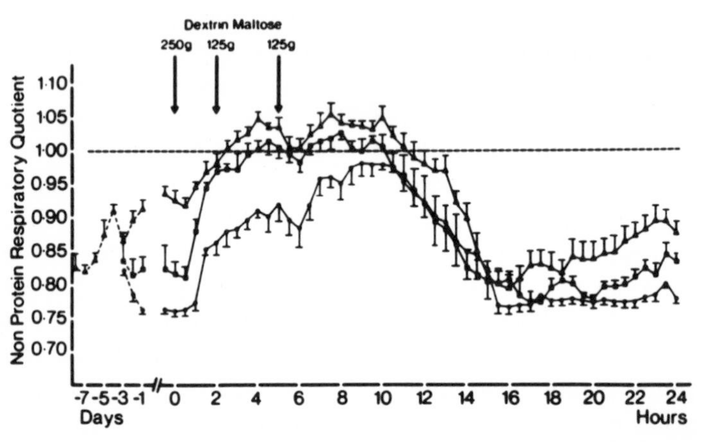

Fig. 1. Changes in the post-absorptive NP-RQ each morning while subjects were on controlled diets (▲ high carbohydrate, ■ mixed, ● high fat), and time course of the NP-RQ during one day in which 500 g of dextrin maltose was consumed in the morning. The surface areas above an NP-RQ of 1.0 indicate periods of net *de novo* lipogenesis. Means ± SEM. Reprinted with permission from ref. *13*.

III. RESTING METABOLIC RATE

Basal and resting metabolic rates are closely correlated with an individual's lean body mass, which itself is well correlated with body surface area and body weight. It is now generally accepted that the resting metabolic rate of obese subjects is greater than that of normal subjects of equal height and age, and that this increment is due to the increase in lean body mass associated with an expansion of the adipose tissue mass. Considering that energy requirements for maintenance are higher for obese than for lean subjects, one could argue that obesity is in effect a more energy wasting state than normal. Since energy expenditure is roughly proportional to body weight (*4*), the same interpretation applies when one compares the costs involved in performing physical tasks required in daily life.

Diet-induced thermogenesis (DIT), although including increments in energy expenditure above the resting rate (*i.e.*, the TEF), is a term primarily used to describe increases in resting metabolic rates induced by overeating. DIT is a major mechanism for the dissipation of energy consumed in excess in many experimental animals

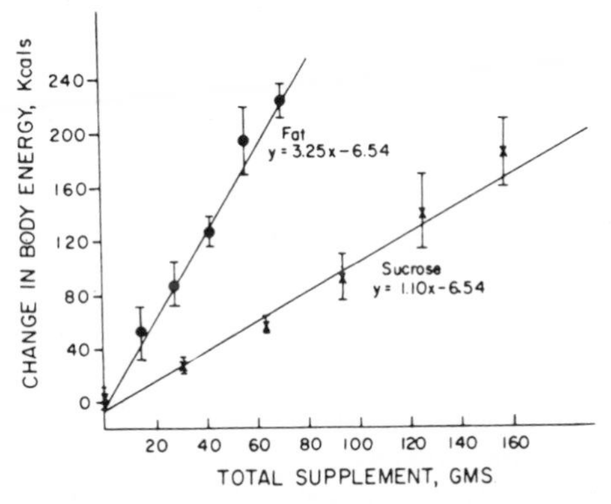

Fig. 2. Change in body energy content of young rats, as a function of amounts of excess fat or excess sucrose consumed over a 21 day period. Reproduced with permission from ref. *17*.

(*15*). It appears to be caused primarily by increased fuel oxidation in brown adipose tissue (BAT), induced by uncoupling of oxidative phosphorylation through activation of a specific proton conducting protein present in the mitochondrial membrane of BAT (*16*). The quantitative importance of such energy dissipation during overfeeding is illustrated by data of Donato and Hegsted (*17*) (Fig. 2) obtained in young rats after 21 days of overfeeding with carbohydrate or fat. The slopes of the lines indicate a retention of only 35% of excess energy consumed as fat, and an even lesser proportion of 28% when the excess energy consumed was in the form of sucrose. On the basis of such findings, these authors have argued that if an intake of 1 g of carbohydrate yields 4 kcal, as proposed by Atwater and Bryand (*18*), then Atwater's value for fat should in fact be 11 rather than 9 kcal/g, at least under conditions of overfeeding. This proposal does not really seem to be tenable, since carbohydrate or fat oxidation will indeed release energy commensurate with their heats of combustions, which average 4.1 and 9.3 kcal/g, respectively. (The Atwater factors are set somewhat lower than these, to account for incomplete absorption of the nutrients.) An explanation for the apparent discrepancy discussed by Donato and Hegsted may be found by considering the metabolic costs incurred for processing different nutrients and the difference in net "ATP yields" which they imply.

IV. ATP YIELDS

The concepts used to explain the process of oxidative phosphorylation have greatly evolved and have led to the realization that the stoichiometry for proton extrusion during the reoxidation of reducing equivalents through the mitochondrial electron transmitter system may, in fact, be variable (*19*). Nevertheless, it has remained general practice to consider that three cytoplasmic ATP's are regenerated per atom-gram of oxygen consumed (*i.e.*, that the P:O ratio is 3 for the reoxidation of 1 mol of mitochondrial NADH). By relating the mols of $ADP+P_i$ converted to ATP during the oxidation of glucose or fatty acids, as predicted from current knowledge of

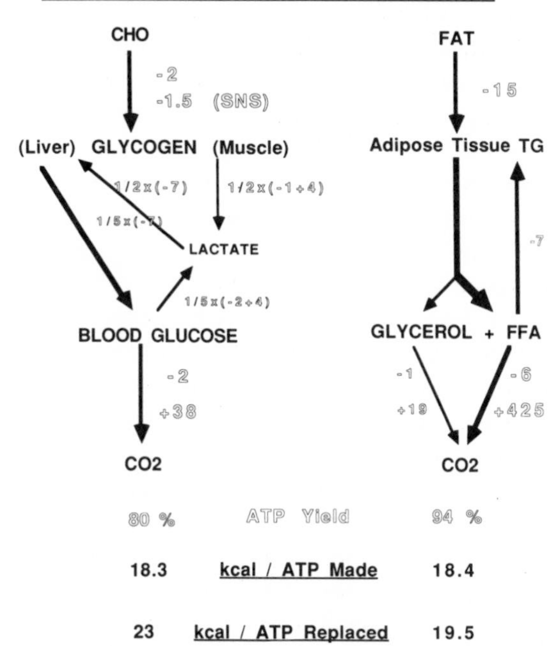

Fig. 3. Scheme describing ATP production (*i.e.*, high energy bond formation) from dietary carbohydrate and dietary fat. The increase in energy expenditure due to stimulation of the sympathetic nervous systems (SNS) is shown by the expenditure of an amount of ATP slightly less than that used for glucose conversion into glycogen. It is assumed that half of the dietary carbohydrate is initially stored in muscle, to be subsequently released as lactate which is then converted into liver glycogen. It is further assumed that 20% of the glucose released from the liver goes through the Cori cycle. In the case of fat, the costs for fatty acid esterification to form chylomicron triglycerides and for subsequent esterification into adipose tissue fat is considered. It is assumed that half of the fatty acids formed by lipolysis in adipose tissue are re-esterified, either directly in this tissue or *via* conversion to very low density lipoprotein in the liver.

metabolic pathways, to the heat of combustion of these substrates, one finds that 18.3 or 18.4 kcal are released per mol of ATP turned over (Fig. 3) (considering that 37 ATP are produced per glucose-moiety of glycogen). The figure shows an approximate estimate of the ATP expenditure associated with the uptake, storage and metabolism of carbohydrate and fat. Because the costs for substrate activation assume greater relative importance for a small molecule such as glucose, as compared to a fatty acid, and because of lactate production and recycling *via* the Cori cycle (estimated here to involve 20% of the glucose metabolized), an amount of ATP equivalent to some 20% of the ATP produced by glucose oxidation may be utilized for these processes. In the case of fat, the ATP dissipated for "substrate handling" is equivalent to only 6% of the ATP generated by fatty acid oxidation. Thus ATP yields may be estimated at about 80% in the case of glucose, and at about 94% in the case of fat (Fig. 3). An expenditure of 23 kcal would thus be predicted for each mol of ATP replaced by oxidation of dietary carbohydrate, whereas in the case of fat this value would amount to 19.5 kcal/mol of ATP replaced. This can account, at least in part, for the greater efficiency of energy retention when excess fat rather than excess carbohydrate is consumed. The ratio between the proportions of energy retained from carbohydrate and from fat observed by Donato and Hegsted (*17*) is 28%/35%=0.81, which is quite similar to the ratio of the ATP yields computed in Fig. 3, *i.e.*, 19.5 kcal per ATP/23 kcal per ATP=0.85. This difference in ATP yields could also explain the increased energy retention observed in man during overfeeding with high fat, as compared to high carbohydrate foods (*1*), without the need to invoke *de novo* lipogenesis as a major cause for excess energy dissipation. The latter has not been a satisfactory explanation because lipogenesis in adult man is relatively limited (*13*). Furthermore, it would be applicable only to a minor part of the carbohydrate consumed in excess, since the fat sparing effect of excess carbohydrate allows a greater proportion of the fat supplied by the diet to be retained.

In the case of protein, an expenditure of 5 to 6 mol of ATP is required for the uptake, transport, and conversion into protein of 1 mol of an amino acid mixture. If ingested amino acids are immediately degraded, a similar ATP expenditure is required for transport, gluconeogenesis and ureagenesis. Thus, the predicted obligatory

TEF for protein approaches 25% regardless of the fate of the ingested amino acids (*7*), which is in good agreement with TEF's observed for protein (*2*). Considering that the amino acids incorporated into protein participate in protein turnover, and that they (or an equivalent amount) are subsequently also degraded with glucose and urea production, only about 50 to 60% of the ATP yielded by amino acid degradation is actually available to replace ATP used in the body. In patients receiving a fixed amount of energy by intravenous infusion, but 364 instead of 180 mg of amino acid-N/kg body weight/day, Shaw *et al.* (*20*) observed an increase in energy expenditure of 2.2 kcal/kg body weight/day, equivalent to 45% of the increment in energy provided from amino acids. The level of dietary protein intake thus has an impact on total energy expenditure, of perhaps 20 kcal/day for a 10 g difference in protein intake.

V. INTAKE AND OXIDATION

A slightly different slant in considering nutrient utilization relates to the effectiveness with which they are used for oxidation or rather for long term storage. In *ad libitum* fed mice, we observed that carbohydrate oxidation is proportional to carbohydrate and food intake, whereas fat oxidation is negatively correlated with food and fat intake (Fig. 4). This implies that the regulation of carbohydrate balance and of fat balance are fundamentally different (see Flatt elsewhere in this book). This reflects the fact that greater priority is given to the preservation of carbohydrate balance than to the maintenance of fat or overall energy balances, a necessity in view of the body's limited capacity for storing glycogen. Studies of the regulation of the overall energy balance, in which carbohydrate and fat calories are summed, thus fail to detect the much more refined control phenomena operating to maintain carbohydrate balance, and their possible impact on the regulation of food intake. As shown by the data in Fig. 4, dietary carbohydrate is preferentially utilized for energy production. This involves temporary storage of much of the carbohydrate consumed in the form of glycogen, but avoids the more substantial energy costs associated with carbo-

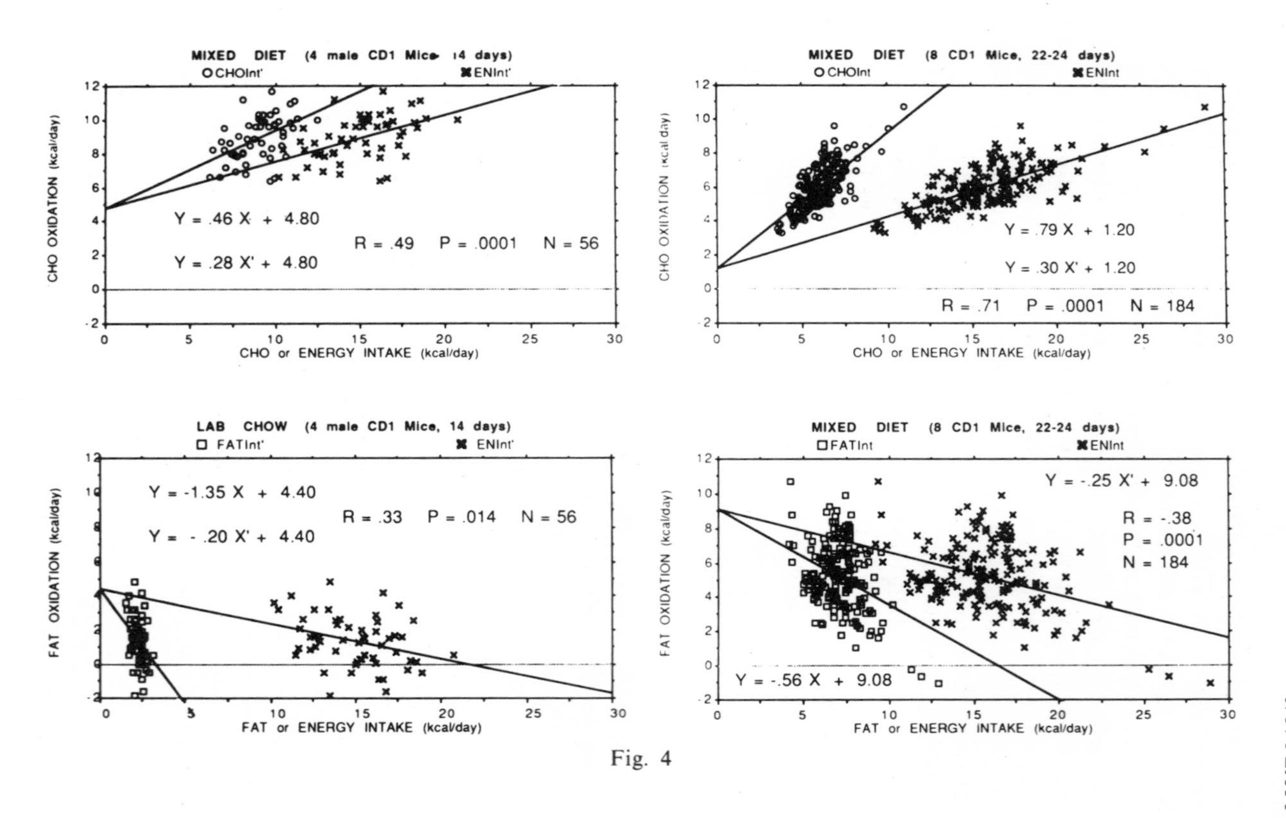
MIXED DIET (4 male CD1 Mice, 14 days)
CHOInt'
ENInt'
Y = .46 X + 4.80
Y = .28 X' + 4.80
R = .49 P = .0001 N = 56
CHO or ENERGY INTAKE (kcal/day)
CHO OXIDATION (kcal/day)
MIXED DIET (8 CD1 Mice, 22-24 days)
CHOInt
ENInt
Y = .79 X + 1.20
Y = .30 X' + 1.20
R = .71 P = .0001 N = 184
CHO or ENERGY INTAKE (kcal/day)
CHO OXIDATION (kcal/day)
LAB CHOW (4 male CD1 Mice, 14 days)
FATInt'
ENInt'
Y = -1.35 X + 4.40
Y = -.20 X' + 4.40
R = .33 P = .014 N = 56
FAT or ENERGY INTAKE (kcal/day)
FAT OXIDATION (kcal/day)
MIXED DIET (8 CD1 Mice, 22-24 days)
FATInt
ENInt
Y = -.25 X' + 9.08
R = -.38
P = .0001
N = 184
Y = -.56 X + 9.08
FAT or ENERGY INTAKE (kcal/day)
FAT OXIDATION (kcal/day)

Fig. 4

hydrate conversion into fat. One also realizes that dietary fat is effectively targeted for deposition and storage in adipose tissue, from which fat withdrawal is determined by the gap between total energy expenditure and energy supplied in the form of dietary carbohydrate plus protein. The amount of fat ingested indeed has no effect on postprandial substrate oxidation (*21*).

The costs incurred for nutrient storage include not only the ATP expenditure required for their initial incorporation into the body's stores, but also the costs for maintaining and moving the tissues which contain these reserves (*22*). The resting metabolic rate increases by about 10 kcal/kg/day of additional body weight. Since the cost of physical activity is roughly proportional to body weight (*4*), a gain of 1 kg causes an increment in energy expenditure of 10 to 15 kcal/day in sedentary individuals. However, for moderately active to physically rather active individuals, these costs will be in the range of 20 to 30 kcal/kg/day (*22*). Thus, it turns out that the degree of physical activity is yet another factor affecting the efficiency with which energy taken in will be retained. It is of interest to note also that the self-correcting effect which changes in body weight exert in compensating for deviations from the energy balance is more powerful in physically active than in sedentary individuals.

In *ad libitum* fed mice, daily energy balances are influenced much more significantly by variations in energy intake than by changes in energy expenditure (Fig. 5). This is because short-term

Fig. 4. Carbohydrate and fat oxidation in relation to carbohydrate, fat and energy intake in *ad libitum* fed mice. Adult CD-1 mice were kept individually in hermetically sealed 55 gal drums, vented once every 24 hr, after measurement of daily CO_2 production and oxygen consumption. Four female and four male mice were followed for 24 or 22 consecutive days, respectively, while provided with a synthetic "mixed diet" containing 18% of its energy as protein, 37% as carbohydrate and 45% as fat. Four other male mice were studied during 14 consecutive days while on lab chow (24% protein, 63% carbohydrate and 13% fat). Daily carbohydrate and fat oxidation were calculated by indirect calorimetry, assuming that the animals maintained an approximately even nitrogen balance. Individual correction factors for food spillage and incomplete nutrient absorption were determined by adding to the cumulated daily CO_2-carbon released 47 mmol of carbon per g of weight change during the entire experiment. The calculations also include individually established correction factors to account for the production of small amounts of hydrogen.

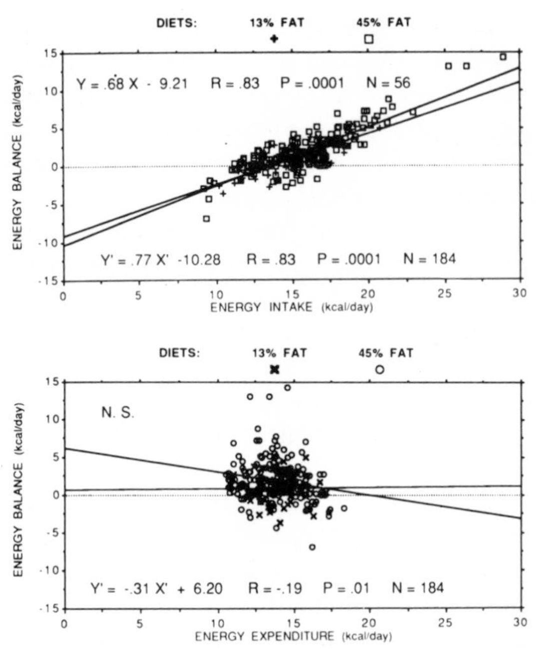

Fig. 5. Energy balance as a function of energy intake and of energy expenditure in 12 *ad libitum* fed mice. For experimental details, see legend to Fig. 4.

changes in energy expenditure brought about by insufficient food intake can only modestly attenuate the energy deficit, or dissipate a minor fraction of the calories consumed in excess. This suggests that adjustment of food intake, whether mediated spontaneously or deliberately imposed, determines whether weight maintenance is achieved or not, whereas factors such as diet composition, exercise habits, metabolic efficiency, inheritance, *etc.* contribute to establish the particular weight for which spontaneous regulation of food intake will tend to promote weight maintenance.

SUMMARY

Metabolic regulation effectively adjusts carbohydrate oxidation to carbohydrate intake, and deviations from the energy balance merely reflect differences between rates of deposition of exogenous fatty acids into adipose tissue and of fat withdrawal therefrom. The high metabolic costs of *de novo* lipogenesis are thereby minimized. But even in the absence of lipogenesis the costs incurred during carbohydrate metabolism exceed those incurred in the metabolism of fat. Thus, net ATP yields during carbohydrate oxidation are estimated at about 80%, whereas ATP yields are likely to approach 95% in the case of fat. To replace a given amount of ATP, a difference in overall energy expenditure of 15 to 20% would thus be expected when dietary carbohydrate or fat provides the metabolic fuel. Based on these estimates, a replacement of 10% of the diet's total energy content with carbohydrate instead of fat would cause a 2% increase in overall energy expenditure. A comparable change in energy expenditure would be caused by a weight gain of 3-4 kg.

Acknowledgments

This work was supported by NIH Grant DK33214. The collaboration of K.E.G. Sargent and B.R. Krauss is gratefully acknowledged.

REFERENCES

1. Sims, E.A.H. (1976). Experimental obesity, dietary induced thermogenesis. *Clin. Endocrinol. Metab.* **5**, 377-395.
2. Kleiber, M. (1975). "The Fire of Life," p. 272 and p. 309. Krieger, New York.
3. Pahud, P., Ravussin, E., and Jéquier, E. (1980). Energy expenditure during oxygen deficit period of submaximal exercise in man. *J. Appl. Physiol.* **48**, 770-775.
4. Pandolfi, K.B., Givoni, B., and Goldberg, R.F. (1977). Predicting energy expenditure with load while standing or walking very slowly. *J. Appl. Physiol.* **43**, 577-581.
5. Segal, K.R., Presta, E., and Gutin, B. (1984). Thermic effect of food during graded exercise in normal weight and obese man. *Am. J. Clin. Nutr.* **40**, 995-1000.
6. Acheson, K.J., Ravussin, E., Wahren, J., and Jéquier, E. (1984). Thermic effect of glucose in man. Obligatory and facultative thermogenesis. *J. Clin. Invest.* **74**, 1572-1580.
7. Flatt, J.P. (1978). The biochemistry of energy expenditure. *In* "Recent Advances in Obesity Research," Bray, G.A., ed., Vol. 2, pp. 211-228. Newman, Washington,

D.C.

8. Welle, S., Lilavivat, U., and Campbell, R.G. (1981). Thermic effect of feeding in man: Increased plasma norepinephrine levels following glucose but not protein or fat consumption. *Metabolism* **30**, 953–958.
9. LeBlanc, J. and Brondel, L. (1985). Role of palatability on meal-induced thermogenesis in human subjects. *Am. J. Physiol.* **248**, E333–E336.
10. LeBlanc, J., Cabanac, M., and Samson, P. (1986). Reduced post-prandial heat production with gavage as compared with meal feeding in human subjects. *Am. J. Physiol.* **245**, E95–E101.
11. Bessard, T., Schutz, Y., and Jéquier, E. (1983). Energy expenditure and postprandial thermogenesis in obese women before and after weight loss. *Am. J. Clin. Nutr.* **38**, 680–693.
12. Acheson, K.J., Schutz, Y., Bessard, T., Anantharaman, K., Flatt, J.P., and Jéquier, E. Glycogen storage capacity and *de novo* lipogenesis during massive carbohydrate overfeeding in man. *Am. J. Clin. Nutr.* **48**, 240–247 (1988).
13. Acheson, K.J., Schutz, Y., Bessard, T., Ravussin, E., Jéquier, E., and Flatt, J.P. (1984). Nutritional influences on lipogenesis and thermogenesis after a carbohydrate meal. *Am. J. Physiol.* **246**, E62–E70.
14. Hultman, E. and Nilsson, L.H. (1975). Factors influencing carbohydrate metabolism in man. *Nutr. Metabol.* **18** (Suppl. 1), 45–69.
15. Rothwell, N.J. and Stock, M.J. (1981). Regulation of energy balance. *Annu. Rev. Nutr.* **1**, 235–256.
16. Seydoux, J., Trimble, E.R., Bouillard, F., Assimacopoulos-Jeannet, F., Bas, S., Ricquier, D., Giacobino, J.P., and Girardier, L. (1984). Modulation of β-oxidation and protein conductance pathway of brown adipose tissue in hypo- and hyperinsulinic states. *FEBS Lett.* **166**, 141–145.
17. Donato, K. and Hegsted, D.M. (1985). Efficiency of utilization of various sources of energy for growth. *Proc. Natl. Acad. Sci. U.S.A.* **82**, 4866–4870.
18. Atwater, W.D. and Bryand, A.P. (1980). *In* "Connecticut (Storrs) Agricultural Experiment Station," 12th Annual Report, Storrs, CT, pp. 73–123.
19. Murphy, M.P. and Brand, M.D. (1987). Variable stoichiometry of proton pumping by the mitochondrial respiratory chain. *Nature* **329**, 170–172.
20. Shaw, S.N., Elwyn, D.H., Askanazi, J., Iles, M., Schwartz, Y., and Kinney, J.M. (1983). Effects of increasing nitrogen intake on nitrogen balance and energy expenditure in nutritionally depleted patients receiving parenteral nutrition. *Am. J. Clin. Nutr.* **37**, 930–940.
21. Flatt, J.P., Ravussin, E., Acheson, K.J., and Jéquier, E. (1985). Effects of dietary fat on post-prandial substrate oxidation and on carbohydrate and fat balances. *J. Clin. Invest.* **76**, 1019–1024.
22. Flatt, J.P. (1983). The metabolic costs of nutrient storage. *J. Obesity Weight Regul.* **2**, 5–18.

Diet and Obesity, Bray, G.A. et al., eds., pp. 101–112.
Japan Sci. Soc. Press, Tokyo/S. Karger, Basel (1988)

Obesity and Taste Preferences for Sweetness and Fat

ADAM DREWNOWSKI

Human Nutrition Program, School of Public Health and Department of Psychiatry, Medical School, The University of Michigan, Ann Arbor, MI 48109, U.S.A.

The development of obesity has often been linked with compulsive overeating of good-tasting foods, particularly sweets and desserts. To the obese, it is claimed "many of the most attractive, almost irresistible foods are those that are rich in carbohydrates, especially sugar" (*1*). Obese persons are said to overeat ice cream, chocolate, and rich desserts because of an elevated preference for sweet taste, sometimes known as a "sweet tooth." In some cases at least, the sweet tooth may have a physiological basis (*2, 3*). Compulsive overeating of sweet desserts has been linked to abnormal functioning of the endogenous opioid system, thought to mediate the pleasure response to sweet taste (*2*). Animal studies have shown that opioid agonists increase the consumption of palatable diets, while opioid antagonists suppress intake and prevent dietary-induced obesity in the rat (*2*). Another hypothesis is that many obese patients suffer from an imbalance of a central neurotransmitter serotonin, resorting to sweet carbohydrates as a form of self-medication (*4*). Since sugar and starch reportedly elevate brain serotonin levels, obese "carbohydrate cravers" are said to overconsume sugar-laden snacks in an attempt to dispel depression and promote a sense of well-being (*3, 4*).

What factors account for the obese patients' preferences for calorie-dense sweet desserts? The notion that craving for sweet carbohydrates is purely a reflection of serotonin imbalance and is independent of taste factors does not appear to be the answer. Specific taste and food preferences are clearly involved. Obese carbohydrate cravers seldom if ever report cravings for apples, corn or potatoes—all excellent sources of dietary carbohydrate. Instead, such "cravers" tend to select ice cream, chocolate candy, pastries, cookies, and other desserts (*3–5*). These foods are not simply carbohydrates: they are most often combinations of sugar and fat (*5*).

It is not surprising that many obese patients prefer such foods over bland starch and fiber. Foods containing mixtures of sugar and fat are among the most palatable in the Western diet. Chocolate candy and ice cream derive between 80% and 98% of total calories from sugar and fat. The fat content of food often plays an important sensory role. While sugar levels are often fixed (16% sugar content for most ice creams), product acceptability may be directly linked to its fat content: premium ice creams contain between 16–18% butter fat as opposed to 10–12% for lower-grade products. The creaminess, richness, and the desirable "mouthfeel" of good ice cream are all functions of its relatively high fat content. Sensory studies have shown that mixtures of fat and sugar are extremely palatable to obese and normal-weight persons alike (*6, 7*).

Mixtures of sugar and fat not only have unique hedonic properties; they appear to be uniquely fattening. Dietary obesity in laboratory animals is most effectively induced by feeding them mixtures of sugar and fat. Obesity promoting diets consisting of sweetened condensed milk and chocolate chip cookies are often used in preference to 32% sucrose solutions or Crisco oil given in addition to the regular laboratory chow. Recent studies (*8*) further indicate that the development of obesity may be influenced by the timing of ingestions of sugar and fat. Rats given fat and sugar in a single meal deposited more body fat than animals fed equivalent amounts of fat and sugar on separate occasions (*8*).

I. SENSORY STUDIES

Studies on obesity and taste have only recently addressed this interaction between sugar and fat (*9, 10*). Early laboratory studies have focused almost exclusively on the study of sugar solutions in water (*11*). Such studies have failed to provide evidence that obese patients over-respond to the taste of intensely sweet sugar solutions (*11, 12*). While some investigators reported increased liking for sweetness among moderately obese subjects (*13*), others have not found any consistent relationship between sweet taste preferences and overweight (*12, 14–16*), or actually showed that severely obese patients disliked the taste of sweet solutions (*11*). Large-scale consumer studies have found no relationship between body weight and sensory preferences for sugar in apricot nectar, canned peaches, lemonade, or vanilla ice cream (*17, 18*).

This apparent disagreement between early laboratory data and persistent reports of sugar or carbohydrate craving in human obesity may have been due in part to subject selection bias. It is often forgotten that obese populations tend to be very heterogeneous. Obesity is now recognized as a multifactorial disorder, with multiple antecedents and predisposing factors, including a range of biologi-

TABLE I
Subcategories of Human Obesity

Diagnostic criteria	Possible options		
	I	II	III
Family history	Neither parent obese	One parent obese	Both parents obese
Age of onset	Adult >20 yrs	Juvenile 10–20 yrs	Childhood <10 yrs
Overweight	Mild 120–150% IBW	Moderate 150–200% IBW	Massive >200% IBW
Excess fat	Mild	Moderate	Massive
Fat distribution	Lower body	Upper body	
Body weight status	Net loss	Stable	Weight gain
Weight cycling	None	1–3 cycles	>3 cycles

cal, psychological, and sociocultural variables. The principal criteria for the classification of human obesities have included the degree of overweight, age of onset, adipose tissue morphology, and the distribution of body fat. Given the broad range of human obesities (summarized in Table I), there is no reason to expect all obese persons to share a single "obese" taste profile or exhibit comparable patterns of food acceptance and diet selection.

Another issue concerns the large variability of individual response. Sensory evaluation studies always distinguish between measures of stimulus intensity and measures of hedonic preference (*19*). Estimates of sweetness intensity, most often obtained using the standard category scale procedure, rise monotonically as a function of sugar concentration (C):

$$I = a_0 + a_1(\log C)$$

and inter-subject variability is low. In contrast, preference (hedonic) functions for sweetness typically increase with sugar concentration, reaching a maximum at an ideal point or "breakpoint". Preference functions then decline as the intensely sweet stimuli are viewed as increasingly less pleasant, and the "average" hedonic function generally follows an inverted-U pattern (*6, 20*). There is a great deal of individual variation. Several studies on obesity and taste have documented that individual differences in hedonic preference are typically far greater than any observed difference between obese patients and normal-weight controls (*16*).

Not surprisingly, a variety of hedonic responses to sweetness have been observed among both obese and non-obese subjects (*15, 18*). Response profiles were initially classified into Type I (rise and decline) and Type II responses (rise and plateau). Recent additions (*16*) include a Type III response (monotonic decline) and a Type IV response characterized by no change at all. These options are summarized in Fig. 1. The inverted-U shape of the mean hedonic function for sweetness may be a composite of divergent individual responses to sweet taste.

The third issue concerns stimulus selection. Past studies on obesity and taste preferences have relied too often on sweet solu-

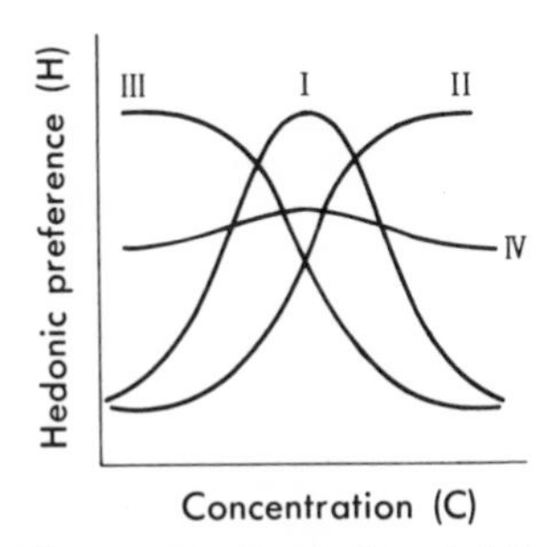

Fig. 1. Idealized plot of different types of hedonic response to sweetness as a function of increasing sugar concentration.

tions, without addressing the obese preferences for sugar and fat. It is important to examine individual responses to complex stimuli that bear at least some resemblance to real foods. In our recent work, we have used mathematical modelling techniques to monitor individual patterns of sensory preference for realistic mixtures of sugar and fat (*5–7, 9*) among clinical populations of women at extremes of body weight.

II. PREFERENCES FOR SUGAR AND FAT

Sensory preferences for mixtures of milk, cream, and sugar were examined in groups of obese women enrolled in a weight reduction clinic, stable reduced-obese women and age-matched normal-weight controls (*9*). A second clinical population at the other extreme of body weight included young women with anorexia nervosa and bulimia, and normal-weight female controls (*19*). Subject characteristics are summarized in Table II.

The patient population spanned an exceptionally wide range of body weights. Values of the body mass index (BMI = weight/height^2), used here as a simple measure of body fatness ranged between 10 and 50. For comparison purposes, BMI values between 18.0 and 24.0 usually indicate normal weight, while BMI of 21.0 represents the median value for young women in the U.S.

Sensory stimuli were dairy products of variable fat content,

TABLE II
Subject Characteristics

	N	Age (yrs)	Weight (kg)	BMI (kg/m^2)
Obese	12	38.0	95.8	34.4
Reduced obese	8	32.7	67.9	23.6
Normal-weight	15	30.1	58.8	21.6
Normal-weight	16	19.1	57.7	21.1
Bulimic	7	19.4	56.8	21.3
Anorectic	25	17.2	40.5	15.5

From refs. *6* and *8*.

TABLE III
Summary of Experimental Design

	Fat g per 100 g	Sucrose levels (% weight/weight)			
Skim milk	0.1	0	5	10	20
Milk	3.5	0	5	10	20
Half and half	11.7	0	5	10	20
Heavy cream	37.6	0	5	10	20
Cream and oil	52.6	0	5	10	20

sweetened with 0, 5, 10, or 20% sucrose weight by weight. The full factorial design (summarized in Table III) provided 20 different mixtures of milk, cream, and sugar. All stimuli were presented chilled to 5 degrees in small plastic cups in a random order. Subjects used the standard sip-and-spit technique and rated each stimulus in turn for its sweetness, creaminess, and the perceived fat content. The subjects also rated their hedonic preference for each item using a 9 point category scale.

There were no differences between obese, normal weight or anorectic subjects in rating sweetness intensity of the stimuli. In contrast, hedonic preference ratings did differ among subject groups. Taste preference responses of obese women patients for mixtures of sugar and fat are summarized in Fig. 2. The standard sucrose breakpoint was obtained for each level of fat, from skim milk to heavy cream. Hedonic preferences also rose with increasing fat content of the stimuli. Obese women who disliked stimuli composed

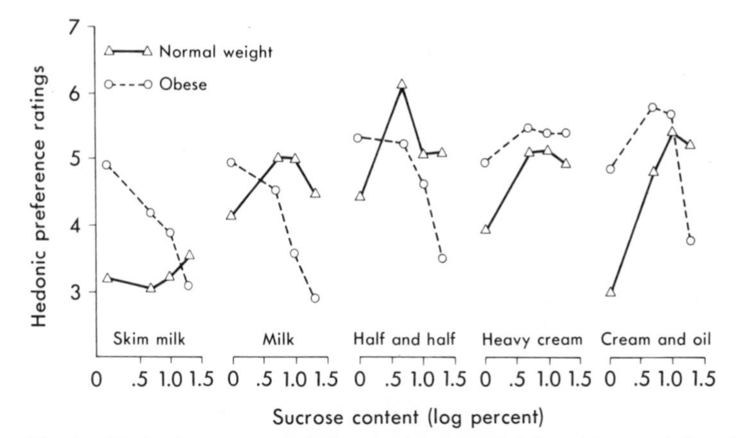

Fig. 2. Hedonic responses of obese and normal weight subjects as a function of increasing sucrose content, shown separately for each level of dairy fat. Sucrose levels are expressed as log percent weight/weight. Data from ref. *6*.

of sucrose dissolved in skim milk showed elevated preferences for equally sweet stimuli consisting of sucrose and heavy cream (*9*).

Sweet taste preferences of anorectic women were also influenced by stimulus fat levels. However, the observed effect was in the opposite direction: hedonic preferences for mixtures of sugar and fat declined sharply as a function of increasing fat content (*19*).

Ingredient composition of mixtures rated as best-tasting by individual subjects was derived using a mathematical technique known as the response surface method (RSM). The present model (*9, 10, 19*) assumes that the hedonic response (H) is a function of both sucrose (S) and fat (F) levels such that:

$$H = a_0 + a_1(\log S) + a_2(\log F) + a_3(\log S)^2 + a_4(\log F)^2 + a_5(\log S)(\log F)$$

After coefficient values a_0 through a_5 were determined, the algorithm was used to predict hedonic responses to a range of sugar and fat levels, including those not actually tested. The model interpolates a number of predicted data points among the 20 empirically obtained ones to create a more accurate representation of the

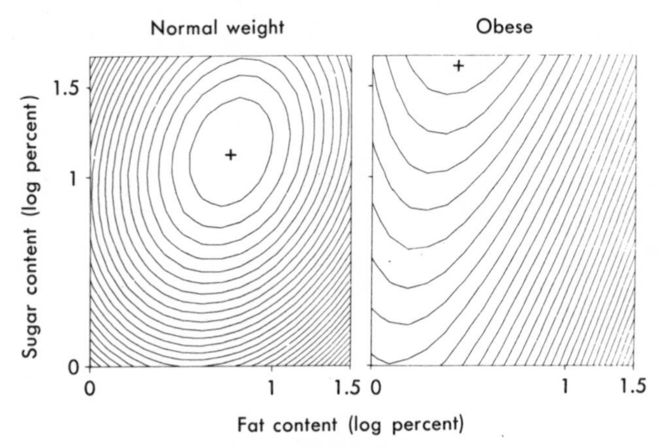

Fig. 3. Hedonic responses of obese and normal weight subjects expressed as isohedonic contours. Sucrose levels (x-axis) and fat levels (y-axis) are shown as log percent wt/wt. The regions of optimum preference are denoted by '+' signs. Data from ref. *6*.

TABLE IV
Optimal Stimulus Composition

	N	Age (yrs)	Sucrose (%)	Fat (%)
Obese	12	38.0	4.4	34.5
Reduced obese	8	32.7	10.1	35.1
Normal-weight	15	30.1	7.7	20.7
Normal-weight	16	19.1	9.1	28.7
Bulimic	7	19.4	15.3	27.9
Anorectic	25	17.2	12.7	16.5

From refs. *6* and *8*.

hedonic response surface than could be obtained from the experimental data alone. A representation of the hedonic surface expressed in the form of isohedonic contours is shown in Fig. 3. The areas of optimum response are denoted by "+" signs.

In our studies, RSM was used to derive optimal sucrose and fat levels for individual subjects. These data were then averaged across subject groups, and means and standard errors are summarized in Table IV.

Obese patients as a group preferred stimuli that were lower in sugar (4% sucrose w/w) but higher in fat content (34% fat w/w) than those best-liked by normal-weight controls. In contrast, anorectic subjects showed highest preferences for stimuli that were sweeter (13% sucrose w/w) but lower in fat (16% fat w/w) than those preferred by their control group (*9*). The present studies indicate that relative preferences for sweetness *versus* fat content may vary inversely as a function of overweight: obese women preferred high-fat stimuli over those that were intensely sweet, while anorectic women craved sweetness but showed a dislike for the oral sensation of butterfat (*19*).

Figure 4 shows a negative relationship between hedonic responsiveness to sweet taste (expressed as the optimal sugar/fat ratio)

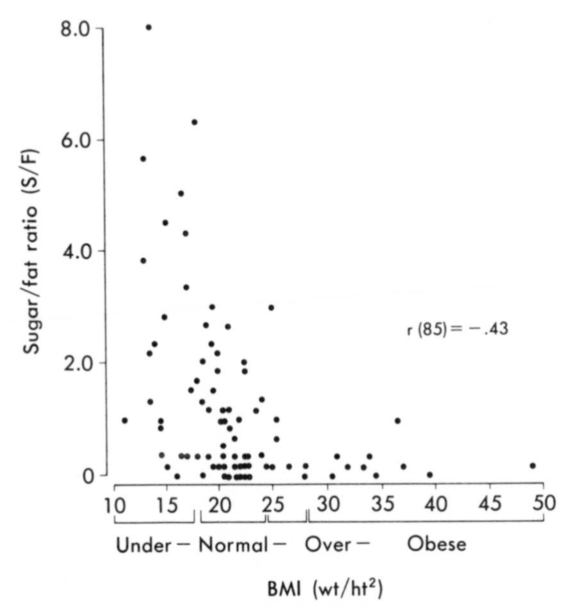

Fig. 4. Relationship between the optimally preferred sugar/fat ratios and body mass indices of anorectic, normal weight and obese subjects. Low sugar/fat ratios denote prefences for fat over sugar in stimulus mixtures, while high ratios denote preferences for sugar over fat.

and the degree of overweight expressed in terms of the body mass index ($r = -0.43$).

However, although statistically significant, this correlation accounted for less than 20% of the variance. Measures of metabolic status other than the degree of overweight may need to be developed to link taste responsiveness with physiological variables, and these additional factors are currently under investigation.

III. CONCLUSION

Hedonic responsiveness to sugar and fat is strongly influenced by the proportions of the two ingredients in the stimulus mixture. Together, sugar and fat exert a synergistic effect on the pleasure response, being much more palatable in combination rather than alone. Sensory studies have also shown that the hedonic response to mixtures of sugar and fat can vary across subjects. Our clinic patients at extremes of body weight followed this general pattern of response: anorectic women showed a liking for sweet taste, while obese women preferred stimuli with elevated fat content.

According to several reports (*3, 4*), starches and desserts figure prominently in the diet of obese women. However, a closer analysis of such "carbohydrate-rich" foods suggests that they are in reality mixtures of sugar and fat (*5*). The sensory role of sugar-fat mixtures in relation to food preference and intake of fat calories in the obese deserves further study. Preliminary studies indicate that the individual patterns of taste preference are remarkably persistent even following substantial changes in body weight. Taste preference profiles of anorectic women did not change following nutritional rehabilitation and weight regain (*19*). Taste response profiles of obese men and women did not change following up to 6 months on a 600 kcal/day diet and very substantial weight loss (between 34 and 43 kg). It may be that individual profiles of taste responsiveness represent a stable individual trait and can be used as an early psychobiological marker for the development of obesity.

SUMMARY

Obesity is often thought to be caused by overeating of good-tasting foods, particularly sweets. Sensory preferences for sweet taste (commonly known as "sweet tooth") are said to be one reason why so many obese women crave sugary carbohydrate-rich foods. However, many popular foods including ice cream, chocolate, and other desserts are not simply carbohydrates: they are predominantly mixtures of sugar and fat. Sensory studies have shown that such mixtures may be especially appealing to the obese. In preference studies with mixtures of milk, cream, and sugar, massively obese women preferred moderately sweet high-fat stimuli over those that were intensely sweet but low in fat content. In contrast, emaciated young women suffering from anorexia nervosa craved sweetness but showed a dislike for the oral sensation of fats. These taste responses appear resistant to short term changes in body-weight, and may serve as an early psychobiological marker for obesity or eating disorders.

REFERENCES

1. Yudkin, J. (1973). The low carbohydrate diet. *In* "Obesity," Butland, W.L., Samuel, P.D., and Yudkin, J., eds. Churchill Livingstone, Edinburgh.
2. Blass, E.M. (1987). Opioids, sugar and the inherent taste of sweet: Broad motivational implications. *In* "Sweetness," Dobbing, J., ed., ILSI-Nutrition Foundation Symposium, pp. 115–124. Springer-Verlag, Berlin.
3. Wurtman, J.J., Wurtman, R.J., Growdon, P., Henry, P., Lipscomb, A., and Zeisel, S.H. (1981). Carbohydrate craving in obese people: Suppression by treatments affecting serotoninergic transmission. *Int. J. Eating Disorders* **1**, 2–14.
4. Lieberman, H.R., Wurtman, J.J., and Chew, B. (1986). Changes in mood after carbohydrate consumption among obese individuals. *Am. J. Clin. Nutr.* **44**, 772–778.
5. Drewnowski, A. (1987). Changes in mood after carbohydrate consumption. *Am. J. Clin. Nutr.* **46**, 703.
6. Drewnowski, A. (1987). Sweetness and obesity. *In* "Sweetness," Dobbing, J., ed., ILSI-Nutrition Foundation Symposium, pp. 177–190. Springer-Verlag, Berlin.
7. Drewnowski, A. (1987). Fats and food acceptance: Sensory, hedonic and at-

titudinal aspects. *In* "Food Acceptance and Nutrition," Solms, J., Booth, D.A., Pangborn, R.M., and Raunhardt, eds., pp. 189-204. Academic Press, New York.
8. Suzuki, M. and Tamura, T. (1986). Simultaneous ingestion of fat and sucrose may contribute to development of obesity: A larger body fat accumulation as compared with their separate ingestion. *Fed. Proc.* **45**, A4 (Abs. 1908).
9. Drewnowski, A., Brunzell, J.D., Sande, K.K., Iverius, P.H., and Greenwood, M. R.C. (1985). Sweet tooth reconsidered: Taste responsiveness in human obesity. *Physiol. Behav.* **35**, 617-622.
10. Drewnowski, A. and Greenwood, M.R.C. (1983). Cream and sugar: Human preferences for high-fat foods. *Physiol. Behav.* **30**, 629-633.
11. Grinker, J.A. (1978). Obesity and sweet taste. *Am. J. Clin. Nutr.* **31**, 1078-1087.
12. Underwood, P.J., Belton, J.E., and Hulme, P. (1973). Aversion to sucrose in obesity. *Proc. Nutr. Soc.* **32**, 93A-94A.
13. Cabanac, M. and Duclaux, R. (1970). Obesity: Absence of satiety aversion to sucrose. *Science* **168**, 496-497.
14. Rodin, J., Moskowitz, H.R., and Bray, G.A. (1976). Relationship between obesity, weight loss, and taste responsiveness. *Physiol. Behav.* **17**, 591-597.
15. Thompson, D.A., Moskowitz, H.R., and Campbell, R. (1976). Effects of body weight and food intake on pleasantness ratings for a sweet stimulus. *J. Appl. Psychol.* **41**, 77-83.
16. Witherly, S.A., Panghorn, R.M., and Stern, J. (1980). Gustatory responses and eating duration of obese and lean adults. *Appetite* **1**, 53-63.
17. Pangborn, R.M. and Simone, M. (1985). Body size and sweetness preference. *J. Am. Diet. Assoc.* **34**, 924-928.
18. Pangborn, R.M. (1981). Individuality in responses to sensory stimuli. *In* "Criteria of Food Acceptance: How a Man Chooses What He Eats," Solms, J. and Hall, R.L., eds., p. 177. Foster-Verlag AG, Zurich.
19. Drewnowski, A., Halmi, K.A., Pierce, B., Gibbs, J., and Smith, G.P. (1987). Taste and eating disorders. *Am. J. Clin. Nutr.* **46**, 442-450.
20. Moskowitz, H.R., Kluter, R.A., Westerling, J., and Jacobs, H.L. (1974). Sugar sweetness and pleasantness: Evidence for different psychophysical laws. *Science* **184**, 583-585.

Diet and Obesity, Bray, G.A. et al., eds., pp. 113–119.
Japan Sci. Soc. Press, Tokyo/S. Karger, Basel (1988)

Intake Timing of Fat and Insulinogenic Sugars and Efficiency of Body Fat Accumulation

MASASHIGE SUZUKI AND TOMOHIRO TAMURA

Biochemistry of Exercise and Nutrition, Institute of Health and Sport Sciences, The University of Tsukuba, Tsukuba 305, Japan

I. OBESITY AND INCREASE OF FAT AND SUGAR INTAKE WITH THE WESTERNIZATION OF FOOD HABITS

Among the dietary factors contributing to obesity, in addition to the positive energy balance, the difference in dietary energy composition has also been suggested to alter body fat deposition, even if energy intake remains the same. Namely, the thermic effect of diet, the so-called energy futile system, has been reported to be much lower in a high fat diet than in a high carbohydrate diet (*1*). This seems to be supported by recent evidence indicating that the fat stored in the body comes mainly from dietary fat and not from dietary carbohydrate (*2*). This lower thermic effect of a high fat diet may be important considering the increasing prevalence of obesity in parallel with the westernization of food habits in Japan. That is, the average daily energy consumption has remained almost constant over the past 7 decades, but the dietary energy composition has changed remarkably: carbohydrate has decreased and fat has increased significantly (*3*).

In Japan, excess body fat accumulation became an important nutritional problem around 1975 when the average dietary fat intake reached 25% of the daily total energy intake.

In addition to the dietary changes in energy composition, the simultaneous consumption of fat from meats and dairy products and sugars from sweet foods and drinks has significantly increased with the westernization of food habits (*4*). This may be another important reason for the rise in the prevalence of obesity.

II. DIFFERENT EFFICIENCY OF BODY FAT ACCUMULATION: SIMULTANEOUS OR SEPARATE INGESTION OF FAT AND SUCROSE

Our several animal studies have demonstrated that the efficiency of body fat accumulation from dietary fat is significantly increased when fat is ingested together with sucrose, as compared with the separate ingestion of fat and sucrose (*5*). This is directly related to the insulin action of the lipoprotein lipase in adipose tissue; ingestion of insulinogenic carbohydrates, such as sucrose and glucose, stimulates lipoprotein lipase activity in the adipose tissue (*6*) but inhibits it in heart and skeletal muscle (*7*). This means that insulin opens fully the fat-gate of the adipose tissue, but partly closes the gates of the heart and skeletal muscle (Fig. 1). Therefore, we have hypothesized that dietary fat simultaneously ingested with sucrose may be more efficiently uptaken and stored by the adipose tissue than dietary fat separately ingested from sucrose.

This hypothesis has been confirmed by a 6-month long-term feeding experiment in male and female rats. Two groups of growing rats 5 weeks of age were meal-fed twice a day. One group, termed simultaneous-eaters, was fed a basal diet at 20–21 hr and a high fat-sucrose diet at 8–9 hr. Another group, called separate-eaters, was fed a sucrose diet at 20–21 hr and a high fat diet at 8–9 hr. Both groups were pair-fed to consume the same amounts of energy, fat, sucrose, and other nutrients every day. Table I shows the composition of the diets. During the feeding period, 33 to 41% of total energy consumed was fat and 9 to 9.6% was sucrose in male rats, and 25 to 41% fat and 9 to 10% sucrose in female rats.

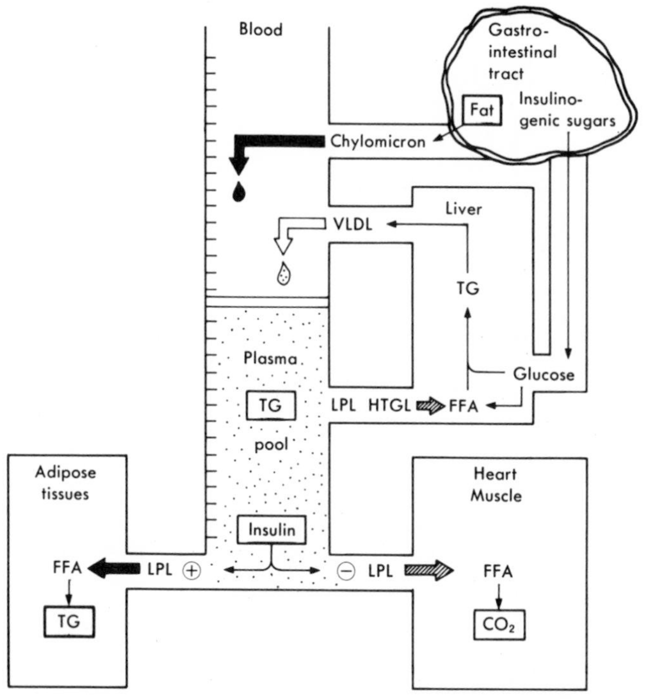

Fig. 1. A proposed mechanism for the increase in efficiency of body fat accumulation by the simultaneous intake of fat and insulinogenic sugars. VLDL, very low density lipoprotein; TG, triglycerides; LPL, lipoprotein lipase; HTGL, hepatic triglyceride lipase; FFA, free fatty acid.

TABLE I
Composition of Basal, High Fat-sucrose, High Fat, and Sucrose Meals (*5*)

	Meals			
	Simultaneous-eaters		Separate-eaters	
	High fat-sucrose (g/100 g diet)	Basal	High fat (g/100 g diet)	Sucrose
Basal (CE-2)	59.3	100	75.0	68.6
Soybean oil	25.7	0	25.0	1.4
Sucrose	15.0	0	0	30.0
	(% of total calories)			
Fat	51.4	11.5	52.6	10.7
Sucrose	12.1	0	0	32.5

TABLE II
Effect of Feeding Timing, Simultaneous or Separate Feeding, of Fat and Sucrose on Body Fat Accumulation in Male and Female Rats Meal-fed Twice a Day for 6 Months (*5*)

	Males		Females	
	Simultaneous-eaters (12)	Separate-eaters (12)	Simultaneous-eaters (12)	Separate-eaters (12)
Mealtimes 08–09 hr / 20–21 hr — Meals	Fat-sucrose / basal	Fat / sucrose	Fat-sucrose / basal	Fat / sucrose
Body weight (g)				
Initial	117±2	117±2	92±2	92±2
Final	512±5	505±9	296±5	286±6
Liver total lipid (mg)	1,520±105	1,635±145	427±15	439±18
(mg/g)	102±7	108±8	51±1	54±2
Adipose tissue (g)				
(Epi/Para+Per+Mes)	39.4±2.5	41.9±2.8	24.7±2.1	21.2±1.7
Carcass (g)	376±5	369±8	204±4	195±5
Carcass fat (g)	100±4*	83±4	48±3*	35±3
(%)	26.4±1.1**	22.6±3.6	23.3±1.4**	17.6±1.3
Carcass protein (g)	60±2	59±2	36±1	35±1
(%)	16.0±0.6	16.1±0.4	17.7±0.6	17.8±0.6

Mean±SEM. ( ), number of rats. *,**Significantly different from separate-eaters (*$p<0.05$, **$p<0.01$). Epi, epididymal; Para, parametrial; Per, perirenal; Mes, mesenteric.

TABLE III
Serum Concentrations of Glucose, Free Fatty Acid (FFA), Triacylglycerol (TG) and Insulin and Lipoprotein Lipase (LPL) Activity in Adipose Tissue, Heart and Skeletal Muscle 3 hr after Consumption of a High Fat-sucrose Meal in Simultaneous-eaters or a High Fat Meal in Separate-eaters (*5*)

	Simultaneous-eaters (6)	Separate-eaters (6)
Serum glucose (mg/100 ml)	159±4	172±4
FFA (μEq/l)	152±19	196±43
TG (mg/100 ml)	188±15**	282±24
Insulin (μU/ml)	22±3*	10±3
LPL activity (μEq FFA/hr/g)		
Epididymal adipose tissue	34.2±3.7*	22.8±2.7
Heart	73.8±8.5	68.7±6.3
Soleus muscle	32.5±7.2	37.7±3.4

Mean±SEM. ( ), number of rats. *,**Significantly different from separate-eaters (*$p<0.05$, **$p<0.01$).

After a 6-month feeding, simultaneous-eaters and separate-eaters in both male and female rats showed similar weight gain, total weight of intra-abdominal adipose tissues and carcass weight (Table II). However, simultaneous-eaters showed significantly larger carcass fat content on both gram basis and percentage expression than separated-eaters of both sexes, basically supporting our hypothesis.

To look at the lipoprotein lipase activity in adipose tissue, male rats 5 weeks of age were divided into the groups described and meal-fed twice a day for 3 weeks on the 4 experimental diets. Animals were sacrificed 3 hr after being fed the high fat-sucrose diet (simultaneous-eaters) or 3 hr after feeding on the high fat diet (separate-eaters).

Simultaneous-eaters showed significantly lower levels of serum triacyglycerols, significantly higher serum insulin levels and significantly higher adipose tissue lipoprotein lipase activity (Table III).

These results suggested that a more efficient body fat accumulation occurred in the animals which simultaneously ingested fat and sucrose, which may be partly due to the more efficient removal of circulating triacylglycerols by the adipose tissue. This assumption was further supported by the data on diurnal changes in serum

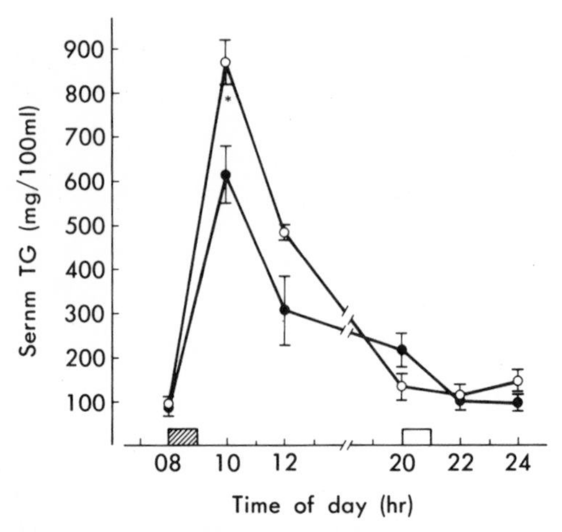

Fig. 2. Diurnal changes in serum triacylglycerol levels in rats meal-fed on high fat-sucrose and basal diets (simultaneous-eaters) and on high fat and sucrose diets (separate-eaters) (*5*). ● simultaneous-eaters; ○ separate-eaters; ▨ fat-sucrose/fat; ▭ basal/sucrose. $^*p<0.05$.

triacylglycerol levels obtained during the feeding period (Fig. 2). Peaks of serum triacylglycerol levels were seen at 1 hr after consumption of the high fat diet in both simultaneous-eaters and separate-eaters, but the levels were significantly lower in simultaneous-eaters. Furthermore, the serum triacylglycerol levels 3 hr after consumption of the fat diet were also considerably lower in simultaneous-eaters.

Thus, our studies demonstrate that the westernization of food habits with their tendency to consume fat and insulinogenic sugar, sucrose, at the same time may be one of the potent causative factors of obesity in industrialized countries. This seems clearly demonstrated by the sample obese subjects studied by Drewnowski (*8*); they prefer high-fat stimuli containing more than 34% fat but less than 5% sucrose while normal weight subjects prefer low-fat stimuli containing a little higher sucrose.

SUMMARY

Animal studies clearly demonstrated that a more efficient body fat accumulation occurs when fat is ingested together with insulinogenic sugar, sucrose, as compared with the separate ingestion of fat and the sugar. This is due to activation of lipoprotein lipase in adipose tissue by insulinogenic sugar concurrently with the increased supply of triacylglycerols into the blood. Thus, westernized food habits in which fat and sugars are usually consumed together may be involved in the increased development of obesity.

REFERENCES

1. Schwartz, R.S., Ravussin, E., Massari, M., O'Connell, M., and Robbins, D.C. (1985). The thermic effect of carbohydrate versus fat feeding in man. *Metabolism* **34**, 285-293.
2. Flatt, J.P. This volume, pp. 87-100.
3. National Nutritional Survey of Japanese. Japanese Ministry of Welfare, Public Health and Medical Affairs Bureau, Department of Health Promotion and Nutrition (1951-1988).
4. Hackett, A.F., Hackett, A.F., Rugg-Gunn, A.J., Appleton, D.R., Allison, M., and Eaton, J.E. (1984). Sugar-eating habits of 405 11- to 14-year old English children. *Br. J. Nutr.* **51**, 347-356.
5. Suzuki, M. and Tamura, T. (1986). Simultaneous ingestion of fat and sucrose may contribute to development of obesity: A larger body fat accumulation as compared with their separate ingestion. *Fed. Proc.* **45**, 481.
6. Eckel, R.H. (1987). Adipose tissue lipoprotein lipase. *In* "Lipoprotein Lipase," Borensztajn, J., ed., pp. 79-132. Evener, Chicago.
7. Borensztajn, J. (1987). Heart and skeletal muscle lipoprotein lipase. *In* "Lipoprotein Lipase," Borensztajn, J., ed., pp. 133-148. Evener, Chicago.
8. Drewnowski, A. This volume, pp. 101-112.

Diet and Obesity, Bray, G.A. et al., eds., pp. 121-128.
Japan Sci. Soc. Press, Tokyo/S. Karger, Basel (1988)

Regulation of Lipoprotein Lipase Activity in Adipose Tissue: Role of Insulin

SHUJI INOUE*1 AND TOSHIO MURASE*2

*The Third Department of Internal Medicine, Yokohama City University, Yokohama 232,*1 and Division of Endocrinology and Metabolism, Department of Medicine, Toranomon Hospital, Tokyo 105,*2 Japan*

Lipoprotein lipase (LPL) is an enzyme which hydrolyzes plasma triglyceride into free fatty acids (FFA) and glycerol, and works for the uptake of plasma triglyceride by the tissue. Adipose tissue LPL permits uptake of plasma triglyceride as storage in fat cells, while muscle LPL utilizes plasma triglyceride as fuel in muscle. Consequently, adipose tissue LPL is very important for fat accumulation.

LPL activity in adipose tissue is regulated by several factors of which insulin seems to be the most important. In this paper, we will demonstrate that insulin regulates LPL activity under various conditions.

By injecting heparin, LPL is released into circulating blood from various tissues, mostly from adipose tissue and muscle. Post-heparin plasma contains at least two lipases: LPL and hepatic triglyceride lipase (H-TGL). We have developed methods of measuring these two lipases separately using specific antiserum prepared against H-TGL (*1*).

I. POSTHEPARIN PLASMA LPL ACTIVITY IN VENTROMEDIAL HYPOTHALAMIC (VMH) LESIONED RATS

Ventromedial hypothalamic (VMH) obesity is produced by lesioning the ventromedial region of the hypothalamus (*2*). VMH lesioned rats are associated with a number of changes, of which hyperinsulinemia is the most characteristic (*3*). Thus, endogenous increase in plasma insulin is produced by VMH lesions.

Using female Sprague-Dawley rats, VMH lesions were produced as previously described (*4*). In the preliminary experiment, we found that blood sampling done 4 min after administration of 200 units/100g of heparin is an optimal condition for measuring postheparin plasma LPL and H-TGL activity (*1*). One week after VMH lesions, 0.7ml of blood was taken from the subclavian venous plexus to measure plasma glucose and insulin under pentobarbital anesthesia; it was again taken 4 min after injection of 200 units/100g of heparin to measure LPL and H-TGL (*5*).

As shown in Fig. 1, VMH lesioned rats fed *ad lib* showed significantly higher postheparin plasma LPL ($p<0.02$) and normal

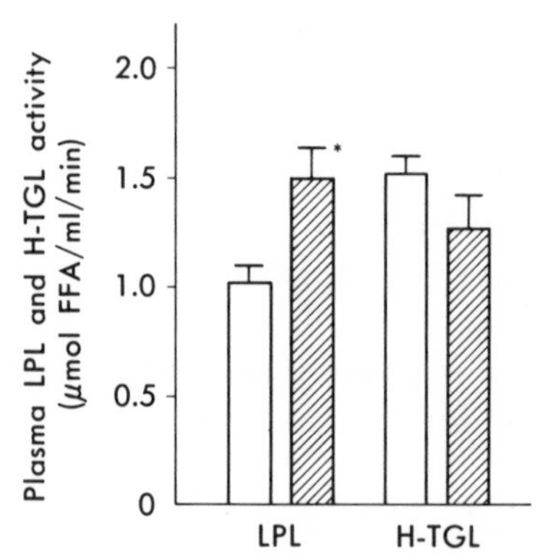

Fig. 1. Postheparin plasma LPL and H-TGL activities in VMH lesioned and sham-VMH lesioned (control) rats fed *ad lib* one week after VMH lesions. ▭ control; ▨ VMH. Values are mean±S.E. $*p<0.02$. Modified from ref. *5*.

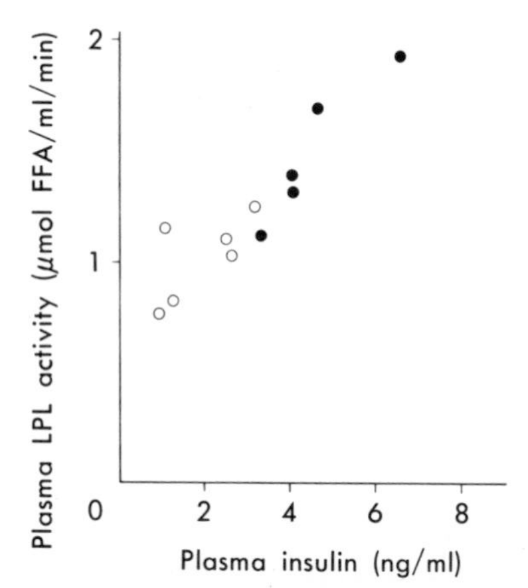

Fig. 2. Relationship between plasma insulin levels and postheparin plasma LPL activity in VMH lesioned and sham-VMH lesioned (control) rats fed *ad lib* one week after VMH lesions. ○ control; ● VMH.

H-TGL activity than sham-VMH lesioned rats. VMH lesioned rats also showed higher plasma insulin levels than sham-VMH lesioned rats (4.54 ± 0.45 *vs.* 1.96 ± 0.39 ng/ml, $p < 0.001$). There was a positive correlation between plasma LPL activity and insulin levels in VMH lesioned rats ($r = 0.947$, $p < 0.02$) (Fig. 2).

According to Tan *et al.* (*6*), about 60% of postheparin LPL activity originates from adipose tissue in normally fed rats. In addition, remarkable increase in body weight after VMH lesions results from increase in body fat (*7, 8*). Consequently, the results suggest that insulin increases adipose tissue LPL. However, there is a possibility that hyperphagia in VMH lesioned rats (*9*) enhances postheparin LPL activity.

In order to exclude the factor of food intake, we did an experiment in an overnight fasting state 1 week after VMH lesions. As shown in Fig. 3, VMH lesioned rats showed significantly higher postheparin plasma LPL ($p < 0.001$) and normal H-TGL activity than sham-VMH lesioned rats. Plasma insulin of VMH lesioned rats was also higher than that of sham-VMH lesioned rats (2.60 ± 0.53 *vs.* 0.76 ± 0.14 ng/ml, $p < 0.02$). There was a positive correlation

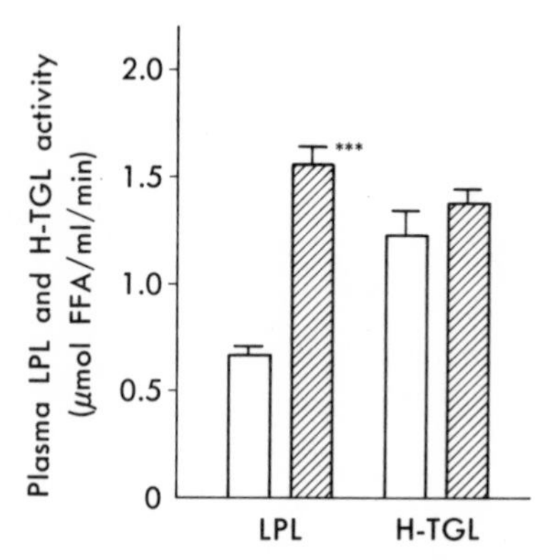

Fig. 3. Postheparin plasma LPL and H-TGL activities in VMH lesioned and sham-VMH lesioned (control) rats after overnight fast one week after VMH lesions. ○ control; ▨ VMH. Values are means±S.E. ***$p<0.001$.

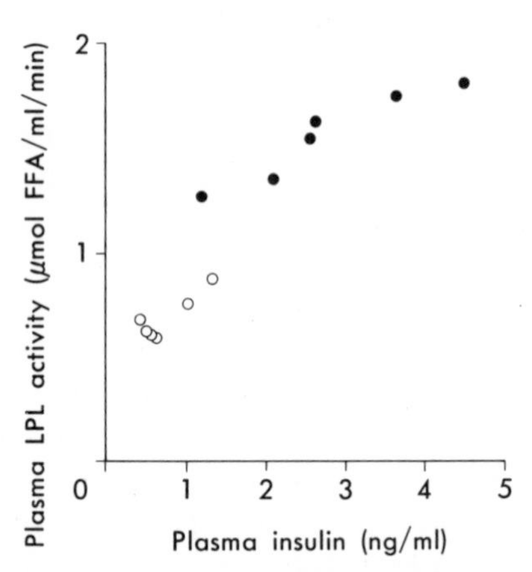

Fig. 4. Relation between plasma insulin levels and postheparin plasma LPL activity in VMH lesioned and sham-VMH lesioned (control) rats after overnight fast one week after VMH lesions. ○ sham-VMH; ● VMH.

between plasma LPL activity and insulin levels in VMH lesioned rats ($r=0.926$, $p<0.01$) (Fig. 4).

It is reported that although adipose tissue LPL activity decreases remarkably, muscle LPL activity does not change after prolonged fasting (6). We infer from this that muscle LPL activity is not insulin dependent. Consequently, we may consider that the elevated part of postheparin LPL activity which is produced by hyperinsulinemia in VMH lesioned rats under fasting condition reflects an increase in adipose tissue LPL activity.

From the results of these two experiments, we may interpret that hyperinsulinemia in VMH lesioned rats increases adipose tissue LPL activity, resulting in acceleration of plasma triglyceride deposition into adipose tissue.

II. POSTHEPARIN PLASMA LPL ACTIVITY IN INSULIN-TREATED RATS

An exogenous increase in plasma insulin was produced by treatment of daily doses of 3 units of insulin (NPH insulin, subcutaneously) for one week. Measurements were done using the same protocol as for VMH lesioned rats. As shown in Fig. 5, insulin treated rats fed *ad lib* showed significantly higher plasma insulin levels and postheparin plasma LPL activity, but normal postheparin plasma H-TGL activity.

The results indicate that insulin increases adipose tissue LPL activity.

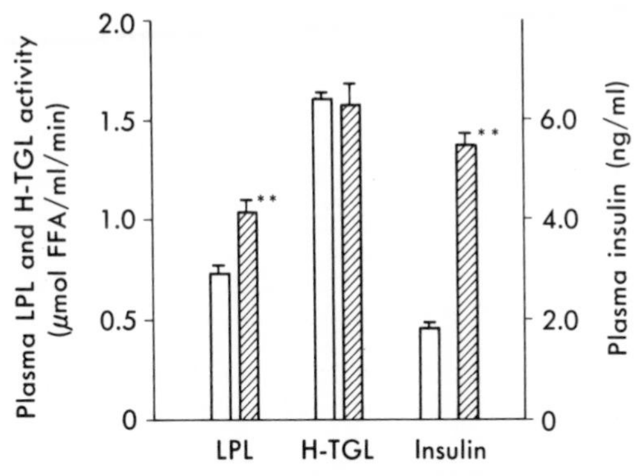

Fig. 5. Postheparin plasma LPL and H-TGL activity, and plasma insulin in insulin treated and control rats fed *ad lib* for one week. ▭ control; ▨ insulin treatment. $^{**}p<0.01$.

III. POSTHEPARIN PLASMA LPL ACTIVITY IN HIGH FAT DIET-INDUCED OBESITY

High fat diet-induced obesity, a model of dietary obesity, is produced by feeding high calorie diet containing a 60% concentration of fat. Plasma insulin of this obesity is in the normal range (*4*). Thus, endogenous normoinsulinemia with obesity is produced by feeding high fat diet for 10 weeks.

Rats with high fat diet-induced obesity fed *ad lib* showed normal postheparin LPL and H-TGL activity, and normal plasma insulin levels (Table I).

The results suggests that obesity *per se* does not increase adipose tissue LPL activity.

IV. POSTHEPARIN PLASMA LPL ACTIVITY IN DIABETIC RATS

An insulin deficient state is produced by administration of streptozotocin (45 mg/kg, intravenously). Measurements were done one week after administration.

Diabetic rats showed lower plasma insulin levels, but normal postheparin plasma LPL and H-TGL activity (Table I).

It is reported that adipose tissue LPL activity decreases while muscle LPL activity increases in insulin deficient rats (*10*). Proba-

TABLE I
Effect of Plasma Insulin on Postheparin Plasma LPL and H-TGL Activity

	Postheparin plasma (μmol FFA·mm^{-1} ml^{-1})		Plasma insulin (ng/ml)
	LPL	H-TOL	
1. Normoinsulinemia with obesity			
High fat diet	0.666±0.180	1.125±0.199	2.27±0.25
Control	0.697±0.156	1.274±0.196	2.38±0.30
2. Insulin deficiency			
Insulin treated	0.653±0.077	1.106±0.122	0.28±0.04*
Control	0.604±0.052	1.194±0.134	1.66±0.10

*$p<0.01$.

bly such increase in muscle LPL activity would compensate low adipose tissue LPL activity, resulting in normal postheparin plasma LPL activity in diabetic rats.

Lowell *et al.* (*11*) demonstrated that rats with hypothalamic knife cuts do not show the increase in adipose tissue LPL activity when hyperinsulinemia is absent, even if they have hyperphagia. Pykalisto *et al.* (*12*) also indicated that a postprandial increase in adipose tissue LPL may result from a rise in insulin secretion because diabetic patients with low insulin response after eating failed to increase adipose tissue LPL with feeding.

SUMMARY

As shown in Fig 6, increase in plasma insulin can enhance adipose tissue LPL activity, while insulin deficiency cannot. Diet can enhance adipose tissue LPL activity if it can stimulate insulin secretion. This enhanced adipose tissue LPL activity accelerates plasma triglyceride deposition into adipose tissue.

On the other hand, increase in plasma insulin inhibits lipolysis by suppressing hormone sensitive lipase in adipose tissue. Both actions of insulin contribute to excessive fat accumulation causing obesity.

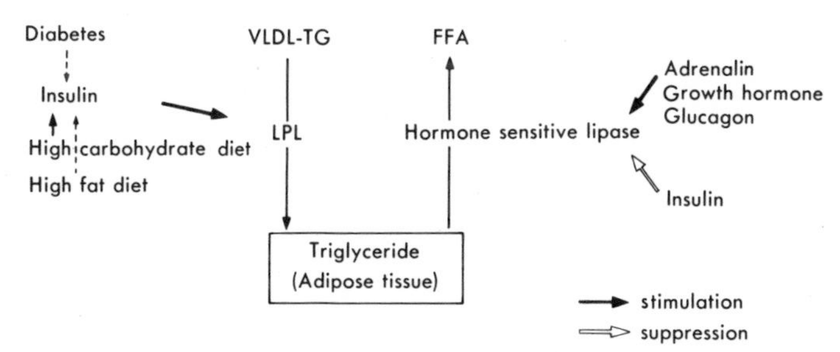

Fig. 6. Schema for insulin action on LPL and hormone sensitive lipase (see text).

REFERENCES

1. Murase, T. and Uchimura, H. (1980). A selective decline of postheparin plasma hepatic triglyceride lipase in hypothyroid rats. *Metabolism* **29**, 797-801.
2. Hetherington. A and Ranson, S.W. (1940). Hypothalamic lesions and adiposity in the rat. *Anat. Rec.* **78**, 149-172.
3. Bray, G.A. and York, D.A. (1979). Hypothalamic and genetic obesity in experimental animals: an autonomic and endocrine hypothesis. *Physiol. Rev.* **59**, 718-809.
4. Inoue, S., Campfield, L.A., and Bray, G.A. (1977). Comparison of metabolic alterations in hypothalamic and high fat diet-induced obesity. *Am. J. Physiol.* **233**, R162-R168.
5. Inoue, S. and Murase, T.(1982). Increase of postheparin plasma-lipoprotein-lipase activity in ventromedial-hypothalamic obesity in rats. *Int. J. Obesity* **6**, 259-266.
6. Tan, M.H., Sata, T. and Havel, R.J. (1977). The significance of lipoprotein lipase in rat skeletal muscles. *J. Lipid Res.* **18**, 363-370.
7. Holm, H., Hustvedt, B.E., and Løvø, A. (1973). Protein metabolism in rats with ventromedial hypothalamic lesions. *Metabolism* **22**, 1377-1387.
8. Martin, R.J. and Lamprey, P. (1974). Changes in liver and adipose tissue enzymes and lipogenic activities during the onset of hypothalamic obesity in mice. *Life Sci.* **14**, 1121-1131.
9. Inoue, S. and Bray, G.A. (1980). Role of the autonomic nervous system in the development of ventromedial hypothalamic obesity. *Brain Res. Bull.* **5** (Suppl. 4), 119-125.
10. Kessler, J.I. (1963). Effect of diabetes and insulin on the activity of myocardial and adipose tissue lipoprotein lipase of rats. *J. Clin. Invest.* **42**, 362-367.
11. Lowell, B.B., Wade, G.N., Gray, J.N., Gold, R.M., and Petrulavage, J. (1980). Adipose tissue lipoprotein lipase activity in rats with obesity-inducing hypothalamic knife cuts. *Physiol. Behav.* **25**, 113-116.
12. Pykalisto, O.J., Smith, P.H., and Brunzell, J.D. (1975). Determinations of human adipose tissue lipoprotein lipase: effect of diabetes and obesity on basal- and diet-induced activity. *J. Clin. Invest.* **56**, 1108-1117.

Diet and Obesity, Bray, G.A. et al., eds., pp. 129–139.
Japan Sci. Soc. Press, Tokyo/S. Karger, Basel (1988)

Diet-induced Thermogenesis, Obesity and Diabetes

LUDWIK J. BUKOWIECKI

Department of Physiology, Laval University, Medical School, Quebec, P. Q., G1K 7P4, Canada

Diet-induced thermogenesis (DIT) represents the increase in energy expenditure observed after a meal. It is usually divided into two major components: obligatory or facultative thermogenesis. Obligatory thermogenesis represents the energy cost of digesting, absorbing and processing nutrients. Facultative thermogenesis mainly appears to be controlled by the activity of the sympathetic nervous system (SNS). Obligatory thermogenesis has previously been called specific dynamic action (SDA) of nutrients. It is generally admitted that a good proportion of DIT can be accounted for by the cost of storing nutrients (*i.e.*, glucose as glycogen or triglycerides, fatty acids as triglycerides, amino acids as proteins or triglycerides). The energy theoretically expended for strong nutrients can be calculated from the ATP requirements of these biosynthetic processes (reviewed by Dr. J.P. Flatt in this book). It has been reported that the measured stimulation of energy expenditure is sometimes higher than the calculated theoretical value (*1*). The difference between the calculated and theoretical value represents facultative DIT. In animals, there is good evidence that the SNS regulates facultative DIT and that a defect in DIT may lead to obesity (*2–4*). Facultative DIT also appears to be modulated by insulin and glucocorticoids that stimulate and inhibit the SNS, respectively (*2*).

I. THE EFFECTS OF HIGH FAT AND HIGH CARBOHYDRATE DIETS ON DIT, OBESITY AND GLUCOSE TOLERANCE

Studies performed with animals have demonstrated that obesity is often linked with hyperinsulinemia, insulin resistance, and a decreased DIT. Considering that insulin activates the SNS (*8*), there may be a direct cause-effect relationship between insulin resistance, a decreased DIT, and obesity (*2*). In our laboratory, we found that hyperphagia induced by liquid sucrose consumption (32%) leads to hyperinsulinemia without compensatory insulin resistance, resulting in an improved glucose tolerance (*19*). It also significantly decreases body weight gain efficiency, possibly by increasing brown adipose tissue (BAT) thermogenic capacity (*21*). On the other hand, hyperphagia induced by palatable high fat diets leads to insulin resistance, a deterioration of glucose tolerance, and an increase in body weight gain efficiency (*9*). It has also been demonstrated that fat (that does not well stimulate insulin secretion) is a more efficient source of body energy than sucrose or protein (which are both potent insulin secretagogues) (*22*). These results support the concept that insulin decreases (and insulin resistance increases) energy gain efficiency, possibly by stimulating DIT in BAT. However, it is likely that the acute effects of insulin are indirect and that they are mediated by the SNS (*8*). Indeed, we have shown that insulin does not directly activate BAT thermogenesis *in vivo* (*23*) or *in vitro* (*24*). Nevertheless, at long term, insulin may regulate BAT thermogenic capacity by controlling mitochondrial protein synthesis (*23*).

In man, the evidence for facultative DIT is scarce and often contradictory. One problem with human studies is that the activity of the SNS is often estimated by measuring plasma catecholamine levels. However, this is not a very sensitive technique since it has been demonstrated that catecholamine turnover may increase in tissues without changes in plasma levels (*5*). To circumvent this problem, several investigators used beta-blocking agents to evaluate the role of the SNS in mediating facultative DIT. While some groups found that propranolol reduced DIT thermogenesis in normal or obese individuals, others did not (*5*). The variations in the composition of the nutrients or the way they are presented (oral intake, intravenous (i.v.) infusions, hyperglycemic-hyperinsulinemic glucose clamps) are often invoked to explain such discrepancies. The palatability of the diet might also represent an important factor modulating DIT (reviewed by Dr. J. LeBlanc in this book).

However, it would appear that, in general, high carbohydrate-low fat meals elicit higher thermogenic responses than high fat-low carbohydrate meals (*6*). This might result from higher increases in obligatory (SDA) and/or facultative DIT induced by carbohydrates. It has also been reported that proteins produced a larger thermogenic response than carbohydrates or fat, but this would mainly be mediated by the greater SDA of proteins (*7*).

II. COLD EXPOSURE REVERSES THE DIABETOGENIC EFFECTS OF HIGH FAT FEEDING AND IMPROVES THE CAPACITY OF RATS FOR DIT

In recent studies, we found that high fat feeding induces hyperinsulinemia and insulin resistance, but only in sedentary warm-acclimated animals (*9*). Cold exposure exerts an "insulin-like" effect on peripheral tissues, reverses the diabetogenic effects of high fat feeding and increases the capacity of animals for DIT (*9–11*) (see Table I for a general summary of the effects of diet composition, cold exposure and exercise training on glucose tolerance and insulin sensitivity).

A possible explanation for the diabetogenic effects of high fat feeding is that an excess supply of triglycerides (and a lack of carbohydrates) in the diet progressively inhibits the activity of the metabolic pathways involved in glucose oxidation as well as in glucose transformation into tryglycerides (Fig. 1). In contrast, high carbohydrate-low fat diets would improve glucose tolerance by stimulating glucose oxidation, and transformation into triglycerides.

More recently, we analyzed the effects of insulin injection (0.5 u/

TABLE I
Summary of the Effects of Exercise Training, Cold Exposure and Diets (High Fat or High Carbohydrate) on Glucose Tolerance, Insulin Response and Apparent Insulin Sensitivity during a Glucose Tolerance Test

Treatments	Glucose tolerance	Insulin response	Apparent insulin sensitivity
High carbohydrate diet	+	++	N/+
High fat diet	−	++	−−
Cold exposure	+	−	++
Exercise training	N/+	−	+
Starvation	N/−	−	N/−
Cold exposure and high fat diet	+	N/−	+
Exercise training and high carbohydrate diet	++	++	+
Cold exposure and starvation	+	−−−	+++

This table summarizes data found in refs. *9, 10,* and *19*. The symbols +, −, and N represent an improvement, a deterioration, or a normal state, respectively. Several identical symbols indicate the relative magnitude of the alterations induced by the treatments compared to sedentary controls living at 23–25°C.

kg i.v.) on the rates of net [^{3}H]2-deoxyglucose uptake (K_I) in peripheral tissues of warm- and cold-exposed animals (48 hr at 4°C). Cold exposure and insulin treatment independently increased K_I values in skeletal muscle (soleus, extensor digitorum longus and vastus lateralis), heart, white adipose tissue subcutaneous, gonadal, and retroperitoneal) and BAT (*12*). The effects of cold exposure were particularly evident in BAT where the K_I increased more than 100 times. When the two treatments were combined (insulin injection in cold exposed rats), it was found that cold exposure synergistically enhanced the maximal insulin responses for glucose uptake in BAT, all white adipose tissue depots and skeletal muscle investigated. The results indicate that cold exposure induces an "insulin-like" effect on K_I which does not appear to be specifically associated with shivering thermogenesis in skeletal muscles, since that effect was observed in all insulin-sensitive tissues. The data also demonstrate that cold exposure significantly potentiates the maximal insulin responses for glucose uptake in the same tissues. Considering that the number of insulin receptors is not usually rate-limiting for the

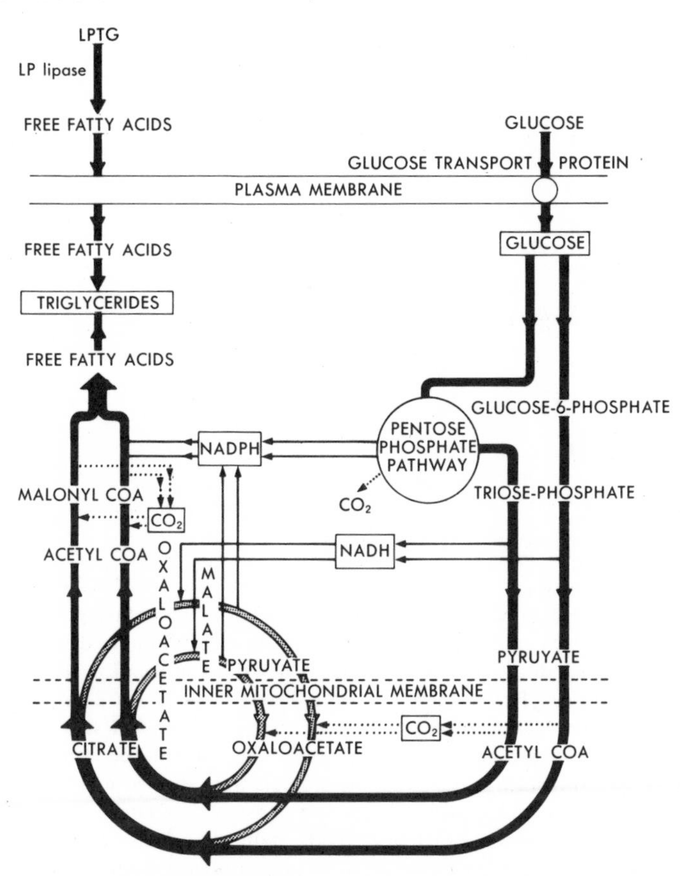

Fig. 1. Metabolic pathways involved in glucose transformation into triglycerides. High carbohydrate diets increase glucose transport, the total number of glucose transporters, the translocation of glucose transporters from a microsomal pool to the plasma membrane (see refs. *14, 15*). High fat diets induce the opposite.

maximal insulin response (*13*), we suggested that cold exposure enhances insulin responsiveness (V_{max}) at metabolic steps lying beyond the insulin receptor (*12*), for instance, at the level of the glucose transport protein (*14–16*). This potentialization may also result from an increase in glucose metabolism consequent to the

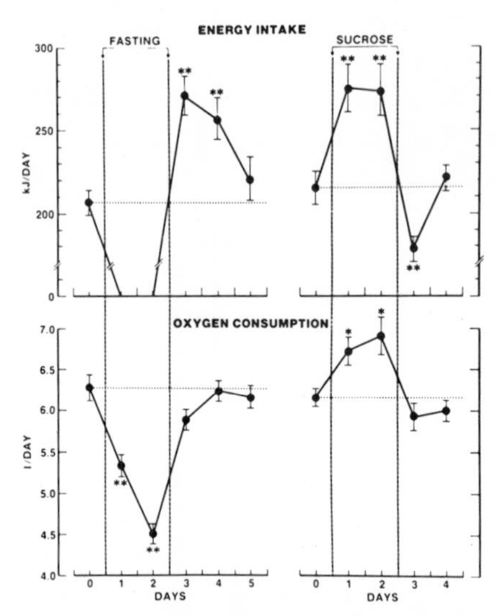

Fig. 2. Comparison of the effects of a 2-day fasting period (left) with a 2-day sucrose overfeeding period (right) on 24-hr energy intake and oxygen consumption. The oxygen consumption system allowing the continuous determination of energy expenditure over several days is described in detail in ref. *20*. Rats had free access to Purina chow and water before and after the 2-day period of fasting or overfeeding. Sucrose was given in the form of 32% solution in the bottles that normally contained water (chow was not removed from the cage). Before the experiment was started, the animals were allowed to adapt to their new cages for at least a week, and oxygen consumption values were recorded 3-4 days before day 0 in order to verify the stability and reproducibility of the measurements. Values are mean -Z⁺ SEM of measurements obtained during 24 hr in 7 rats. Significant differences from control values (day 0) are indicated by (*) ($p<0.05$) and (**) ($p<0.01$). It can be seen that fasting for one day decreased the mean oxygen consumption during the same day by 15% (left). During the second day of fasting, oxygen uptake dropped by an additional 15%. Thereafter, when the rats were fed again, oxygen consumption rapidly returned to basal levels but energy intake increased above pre-fasting values by 20-30% during 2 days, before returning to control values on the third day. Liquid sucrose feeding increased the total energy intake from sucrose and Purina chow by 30% during 2 days (right). It also increased oxygen consumption by 9 and 12% during the first and second day, respectively. Thereafter, when the liquid sucrose was substituted by tap water, a transient, but significant hypophagia occurred during one day. However, oxygen uptake

stimulation of shivering thermogenesis (skeletal muscles) and non-shivering thermogenesis (skeletal muscles, BAT, and other tissues). Our most recent results suggest that the increased nonshivering thermogenesis in skeletal muscles of cold-acclimated rats represents the major phenomenon explaining the reversal of the diabetogenic effects of high fat feeding (*9*).

III. EXERCISE TRAINING IMPROVES GLUCOSE TOLERANCE IN HIGH CARBOHYDRATE FED ANIMALS

Similarly to cold exposure, exercise training decreases circulating plasma insulin levels and increases the apparent sensitivity of peripheral tissues to insulin (see refs. *17, 18*). In recent experiments, we evaluated the interactions between exercise and high carbohydrate feeding (32% sucrose solution and Purina chow *ad libitum*) on glucose tolerance (*19*). Results from these studies indicated that (1) high carbohydrate (sucrose) feeding at room temperature leads to hyperinsulinemia, but contrary to high fat feeding, it improves glucose tolerance without deteriorating insulin sensitivity; (2) exercise training increases the sensitivity of peripheral tissues to insulin; and (3) the marked improvement of glucose tolerance observed in sucrose-trained animals results from a synergistic combination of the above two factors, *i.e.*, increased insulinemia (induced by diet) and enhanced insulin sensitivity (induced by training).

IV. CONCLUSION

The effects of diet composition on DIT are still poorly under-

immediately returned to basal values. The ratio of energy expenditure/energy intake was 21–28% lower during the 2 days following starvation than before starvation ($p < 0.01$), indicating thereby a tendency to conserve energy following calorie deprivation. Likewise, the same ratio was significantly higher after sucrose feeding than before sucrose feeding ($p < 0.01$), showing that energy dissipation relative to energy intake was transiently increased after hyperphagia. Thus, the data show that short-term fasting or hyperphagia induces compensatory alterations of energy balance, not only during but also after treatments. They entirely support the energy buffering concept. For further details see ref. *20*.

stood. However, the use of an oxygen consumption system that continuously records 24-hr energy expenditure in laboratory animals will allow for investigation of the mechanisms of the regulatory alterations in DIT (*20*). Using this system, we were able to show that fasting or overfeeding rapidly induces regulatory alterations in daily energy expenditure. Energy expenditure is decreased, not only during fasting, but also for a few days after fasting. On the contrary, overfeeding stimulates energy expenditure during and after hyperphagia (Fig. 2). This demonstrates the existence of regulatory mechanisms that tend to conserve or dissipate energy expenditure in function of energy intake. The existence of such a buffering system was postulated a long time ago by French scientists who called it "le pondérostat" (literally translated as "body weight-stat") to emphasize the fact that the majority of people maintain a constant body weight throughout life in spite of great daily variations of energy intake and expenditure.

The effects of diet composition and stimulation of energy expenditure by exercise or cold exposure on glucose tolerance and insulin sensitivity are rather well defined. Insulin sensitivity can be improved in laboratory animals by high carbohydrate feeding, exercise training and/or cold exposure. Likewise, insulin sensitivity is deteriorated by feeding high fat diets to sedentary animals living at temperatures close to thermoneutrality (Table I). Taken altogether, the data on laboratory animals would support the suggestion of combining exercise in a cold environment with moderate intake of high carbohydrate diets as a means of controlling the incidence of diabetes and obesity in man.

SUMMARY

The effects of diet composition (high fat *versus* high carbohydrate), exercise and cold exposure on glucose tolerance and DIT in laboratory animals will be briefly reviewed. Long-term high fat feeding in sedentary animals living at room temperature (25°C) leads to hyperinsulinemia, insulin resistance, and a deterioration of glucose tolerance. High carbohydrate feeding (liquid sucrose and

Purina chow) also induces hyperinsulinemia but without compensatory insulin resistance, resulting in an improvement of insulin responsiveness. Although the effects of diet composition on DIT are still poorly defined, it is generally considered that high carbohydrate diets are more thermogenic than high fat diets. Stimulation of energy expenditure by cold exposure (4 °C) or exercise training decreases plasma insulin levels and improves glucose tolerance, suggesting that insulin action on peripheral tissues is increased when energy expenditure is stimulated. Cold exposure reverses the diabetogenic effects of high fat feeding, demonstrating that nutrition-induced insulin resistance is amplified in sedentary animals living at temperatures close to thermoneutrality. Radioactive tracer studies of 2-deoxyglucose uptake in peripheral tissues revealed that cold exposure synergistically potentiates the effects of insulin on glucose uptake in skeletal muscles as well as in white and brown adipose tissues of both warm- and cold-acclimated animals. Thus, cold exposure exerts an "insulin-like effect" on glucose uptake that does not appear to be specifically associated with shivering thermogenesis in skeletal muscles. More recent studies (unpublished) showed that cold exposure improves glucose tolerance and stimulates glucose uptake in starved animals (in the virtual absence of circulating insulin) nearly by the same order of magnitude as in fed animals. It is therefore concluded that cold exposure, and possibly also exercise, improve glucose tolerance and stimulate glucose uptake in peripheral tissues primarily by enhancing glucose oxidation *via* insulin-independent pathways, and secondarily by increasing the responsiveness of peripheral tissues to insulin.

Acknowledgments

This work was supported by grants from the Medical Research Council of Canada and the Canadian Diabetes Association.

REFERENCES

1. Acheson, K.J., Ravussin, E., Wahren, J., and Jequier, E. (1984). Thermic effect of glucose in man, obligatory and facultative thermogenesis. *J. Clin. Invest.* **74**,

1572–1580.

2. Trayhurn, P. (1986). Brown adipose tissue and energy balance. *In* "Brown Adipose Tissue," Trayhurn, P. and Nicholls, D., eds., pp. 299–338. Arnold A. E., London.
3. Rothwell, N.J. and Stock, M.J. (1986). Brown adipose tissue and diet-induced thermogenesis. *In* "Brown Adipose Tissue," Trayhurn, P. and Nicholls, D., eds., pp. 269–298. Arnold A. E., London.
4. Himms-Hagen, J. (1986). Brown adipose tissue and cold-acclimation. *In* "Brown Adipose Tissue," Trayhurn, P. and Nicholls, D., eds., pp. 214–268. Arnold A. E., London.
5. Vernet, O., Nacht, C.-A., Christin, J., Schutz, Y., Danforth, E., and Jequier, E. (1987). Beta-adrenergic blockage and intravenous nutrient-induced thermogenesis in lean and obese women. *Am. J. Physiol.* **253**, E65–E71.
6. Schwartz, R.S., Ravussin, E., Massari, M., O'Connell, M., and Robbins, D.C. (1985). The thermic effect of carbohydrate versus fat feeding in man. *Metabolism* **34**, 285–293.
7. Garrow, J.S. (1985). The contribution of protein synthesis to thermogenesis in man. *Int. J. Obesity* **9**, 97–101.
8. Landsberg, L. and Young, J.B. (1983). Autonomic regulation of thermogenesis. *In* "Mammalian Thermogenesis," Girardier, L. and Stock, M.J., eds., pp. 99–140. Chapman and Hall, London.
9. Vallerand, A., Lupien, J., and Bukowiecki, L.J. (1986). Cold exposure reverses the diabetogenic effects of high-fat feeding. *Diabetes* **35**, 329–334.
10. Vallerand, A., Lupien, J., and Bukowiecki, L.J. (1986). Interactions of cold exposure and starvation on glucose tolerance and insulin response. *Am. J. Physiol.* **245**, E575–E581.
11. Bukowiecki, L.J., Collet, A.J., Follea, N., Guay, G., and Jahjah, L. (1982). Brown adipose tisisue hyperplasia: a fundamental mechanism of adaptation to cold and hyperphagia. *Am. J. Physiol.* **242**, E353–E359.
12. Vallerand, A., Perusse, F., and Bukowiecki, L.J. (1987). Cold exposure potentiates the effect of insulin on *in vivo* glucose uptake. *Am. J. Physiol.* **253**, E179–E186.
13. Olefsky, J.M. (1980). Insulin resistance and insulin action. *Diabetes* **30**, 148–162.
14. Kahn, B.B. and Cushman, S.W. (1986). The glucose transport system: role in insulin action and its perturbation in altered metabolic states. *Diabet. Metab. Rev.* **1**, 203–227.
15. Kahn, B.B., Horton, E.S., and Cushman, S.W. (1987). Mechanism for enhanced glucose transport response to insulin in adipose cells from chronically hyperinsulinemic rats. *J. Clin. Invest.* **79**, 853–858.
16. Kono, T., Robinson, F.W., Blevis, T.L., and Ezaki, O. (1982). Evidence that the translocation of the glucose transport activity is the major mechanism of insulin action of glucose transport in fat cells. *J. Biol. Chem.* **257**, 10942–10947.
17. Richter, E.A., Ruderman, N.B., and Schneider, S.H. (1981). Diabetes and exercise.

Am. J. Med. **70**, 201-209.
18. Horton, E.S. (1986). Exercise and physical training. *Diabet./Metab. Rev.* **2**, 1-17.
19. Vallerand, A., Lupien, J., and Bukowiecki, L.J. (1986). Synergistic improvement of glucose tolerance by sucrose feeding and exercise training. *Am. J. Physiol.* **250**, E607-E614.
20. Shibata, H. and Bukowiecki, L.J. (1987). Regulatory alterations in daily energy expenditure induced by fasting or overfeeding in unrestrained rats. *J. Appl. Physiol.* **63**, 465-470.
21. Bukowiecki, L., Lupien, J., Follea, N., and Jahjah, L. (1983). Effects of sucrose, caffeine, and cola beverages on obesity, cold resistance, and adipose tissue cellularity. *Am. J. Physiol.* **244**, R500-R507.
22. Donato, K. and Hegsted, D.M. (1985). Efficiency of utilization of various sources of energy for growth. *Proc. Natl. Acad. Sci. U.S.A.* **82**, 4866-4870.
23. Shibata, H., Perusse, F., and Bukowiecki, L.J. (1987). The role of insulin in nonshivering thermogenesis. *Can. J. Physiol. Pharmacol.* **65**, 152-158.
24. Bukowiecki, L. (1985). Regulation of energy expenditure in brown adipose tissue. *Int. J. Obesity* **9** (Suppl. 2), 31-42.

PREVENTION OF EXCESS BODY FAT DEPOSITION BY DIETING AND EXERCISE

Diet and Obesity, Bray, G.A. et al., eds., pp. 143-152.
Japan Sci. Soc. Press, Tokyo/S. Karger, Basel (1988)

Comparison of Pathophysiology between Subcutaneous-type and Visceral-type Obesity

SEIICHIRO TARUI, SIGENORI FUJIOKA,
KATSUTO TOKUNAGA, AND YUJI MATSUZAWA

Department of Internal Medicine, Osaka University Medical School, Osaka 553, Japan

I. HETEROGENEITY OF OBESITY

Obesity has been generally defined as excessive storage of energy in the form of fat. Human obesity is, however, heterogeneous from the aspect of topographical distribution of fat in each subject. Android (abdominal, or upper body) obesity and gynoid (peripheral, or lower body) obesity are representative categories of this classification. The frequency of metabolic complications, including glucose intolerance and hyperlipidemia, has been shown to be far more closely related to the former type of obesity than to the latter type (*1-3*). The high waist-hip circumference ratio as representative of abdominal obesity has thus seemed to prove a feasible index in predicting risks associated with fat accumulation. Analyses of the relation between topographical fat distribution and metabolic disorders were done in our laboratory using computed tomography (CT) scanning at various body levels of obese subjects (*4, 5*). As a result, abdominal obesity was still recognized as a heterogeneous condition from the aspect of body fat topography. Abdominal obesity can be further classified into two categories, subcutaneous-type and visceral-type. Most subjects with lower body obesity are of the subcutaneous type, and these two classifications may also be considered applicable to human obesity generally. The close relation between visceral-type obesity and metabolic disorders was shown by data obtained in our laboratory. Anthropological viewpoints on types of obesity are also given in the present paper.

II. ABDOMINAL OBESITY *VS.* PERIPHERAL OBESITY

We first reexamined the classical concept that abdominal obesity is more closely related to metabolic disorders than peripheral obesity, using a modern technique. Fat distribution of obese subjects with 34.1±5.5 kg/m^2 of body mass index (BMI) was determined by CT scan (General Electric CT/T scanner) in the supine position; subcutaneous fat area and intraabdominal visceral fat area were

TABLE I
Metabolic Features of Abdominal Obesity and Peripheral Obesity

	Abdominal obesity	Peripheral obesity
Abdominal fat/femoral fat	≧3	<3
Number of subjects	17	29
Male	8	7
female	9	22
Age (yrs)	52±17	36±17
Duration of obesity (yrs)	19±11	18±11
% IBM	159±22	169±23
Fasting plasma glucose (mg/dl)	125±45	100±35
Plasma glucose area (mg. min/dl)×10^{-2}	385±182*	273±125
Fasting plasma insulin (μU/ml)	14±6	16±8
Plasma insulin area (μU. min/ml)×10^{-2}	104±63	140±79
Total cholesterol (mg/dl)	255±36**	217±30
Triglyceride (mg/dl)	225±104*	154±84
HDL-cholesterol (mg/dl)	44±12	49±15

*$p<0.05$, **$p<0.01$. Mean±SD. Glucose or insulin area: area under the curve on oral glucose (75 g) tolerance test.

measured at the level of the umbilicus and subcutaneous fat area was measured at the midpoint of the thighs.

When the ratio of abdominal fat (subcutaneous fat area plus intraabdominal fat area at the level of the umbilicus)/femoral fat (subcutaneous fat at the midpoint of thighs) is equal to or more than 3.0 in an obese person, the subject is defined as being abdominally obese. Obese subjects whose ratio is less than 3.0 are peripherally obese.

Table I compares metabolic features between abdominal obesity and peripheral obesity. Although the degree of obesity (% ideal body weight, IBW) of these two groups was in the same general range, fasting hyperglycemia, elevated plasma glucose area on oral glucose tolerance test (OGTT), hypercholesterolemia, and hypertriglyceridemia were demonstrated only in abdominal obesity. On the contrary, at least the averages of these metabolic indices were within normal range in peripheral obesity. These studies included subjects of both sexes and the relative frequency of peripheral obesity was higher in females than males, possibly reflecting a so-called sexual dimorphism in *Homo sapiens.*

III. VISCERAL-TYPE OBESITY *VS.* SUBCUTANEOUS-TYPE OBESITY

At least some abdominal obesity is thus demonstrated to be associated with metabolic disorders even through the analyses using the CT scan. However, CT scan imagings have also indicated that abdominal obesity is not a homogenous condition. Figure 1 shows two representative cases with similar abdominal circumference. In the left subject there is little subcutaneous fat; a marked accumulation is observed in the intraabdominal cavity as omental and mesenteric fat. In contrast, fat accumulation occurs exclusively in the subcutis in the right subject. These two cases are extremes of abdominal obesity.

When the ratio of visceral fat/subcutaneous fat at the level of the umbilicus is equal to or more than 0.4, the obesity is defined as visceral-type and when the ratio is less than 0.4, it is defined as subcutaneous-type in the present paper. Metabolic features of the

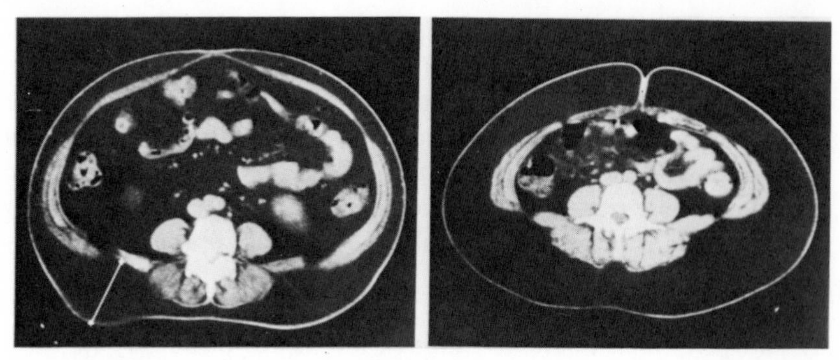

Fig. 1. Two extremes of abdominal obesity: visceral-type (left) and subcutaneous-type (right).

two types are compared in obese subjects of both sexes (Fig. 2). Although deviations from ideal body weight (IBW) are comparable in these two groups, increased plasma glucose area on OGTT, hypertriglyceridemia and hypercholesterolemia were demonstrated only in the visceral-type group. In the subcutaneous-type at least the averages of these parameters were all within normal range. Although the visceral-type group was predominantly male and of relatively higher ages, an age-matched and sex-matched comparison of the two groups showed the same conclusion, indicating that mechanisms specific to the visceral-type are responsible for the occurrence of metabolic disorders beyond the sexual dimorphism.

It is of great importance to learn why visceral fat accumulation causes metabolic disorder. Our previous observations on ventromedial hypothalamus (VMH) lesioned obese rats indicated that mesenteric fat weight is closely correlated with portal free fatty acid (FFA) concentration and fasting plasma glucose level. Metabolites of visceral fat enter the liver directly through portal circulation.

One of the characteristics of mesenteric fat is the marked tendency to become hypertrophic in the obese state. Adipocytes in the intraabdominal cavity are significantly more hypertrophic than those in the subcutis in Zucker (*fa/fa*) rats, although in lean rats mesenteric adipocytes have rather less volume. An increased turnover through rapid biosynthesis and lipolysis could cause excess

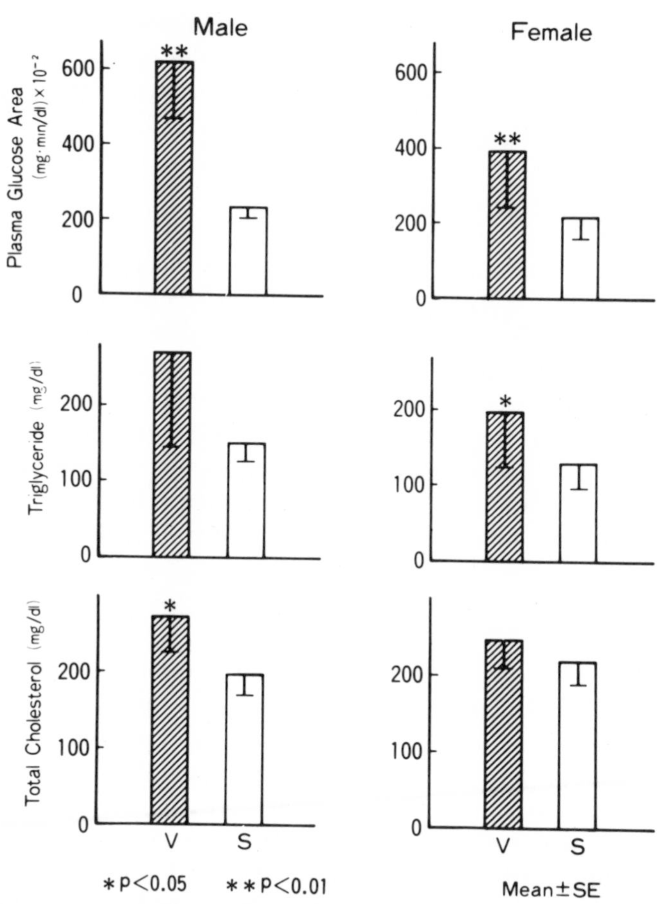

Fig. 2. Comparison of metabolic features between visceral-type and subcutaneous-type obesity. V, visceral-type (8 males and 10 females); S, subcutaneous-type (7 males and 21 females).

efflux of FFA from hypertrophic visceral adipocytes into portal circulation. The excess influx of FFA into the liver might cause an overproduction of very low density lipoprotein, resulting in hypertriglyceridemia and hypercholesterolemia. In regard to carbohydrate metabolism, FFAs have hitherto been shown to inhibit glucokinase activity through the formation of acyl CoA (*6*) and also to affect another key regulatory glycolytic enzyme, phosphofructokinase, either directly (*7*) or through the formation of citric acid (*8, 9*). Glucose utilization could thus be substantially impaired by excess influx of portal FFAs.

IV. ANTHROPOLOGICAL ASPECTS

A more important problem than the biochemical basis for the visceral-type of obesity is what kind of food causes this condition. Contemporary affluent advanced societies provide an increasing number of opportunities for overeating and obesity and a decrease in muscular exercise. There have been arguments about the origin of obesity. Even in ancient societies food scarcities were not necessarily always the norm. In "Gilgamesh," the representative epic written in ancient Sumer, the following expressions were found:

> *"Man, the tallest, cannot reach to heaven. Man, the widest, cannot cover the earth."*
>
> *"I am a lady who wears large garments; I want to cut them."*

Statuettes belonging to prehistoric or ancient societies such as Venus of Willendorf, and Venus of Lespugue (Fig. 3a) show marked fat accumulation in lower segments. Even more marked obesity is demonstrated in the statuette of a nude woman (Fig. 3c) discovered in Turkish territory; it again shows a feature of lower body obesity. The old Japanese rolled book with the name "Yamai-zoshi" illustrated various morbid states. Among them, "a very obese woman who can hardly walk" was painted as shown in Fig. 3b. Although the possibility exists that she was suffering from Cushing's syndrome, it was well known at that time 800 years ago that this type of obesity, upper body obesity, was unhealthy and morbid. Since the ancient statuettes were considered symbols of fertility and fecundity, or at least some graceful happy presence, lower body obesity was apparently not considered unhealthy.

In Japan professional sumo wrestling continues to maintain its popularity as a national sport despite the inroads made recently by professional baseball. Sumo wrestlers are, without exception, very

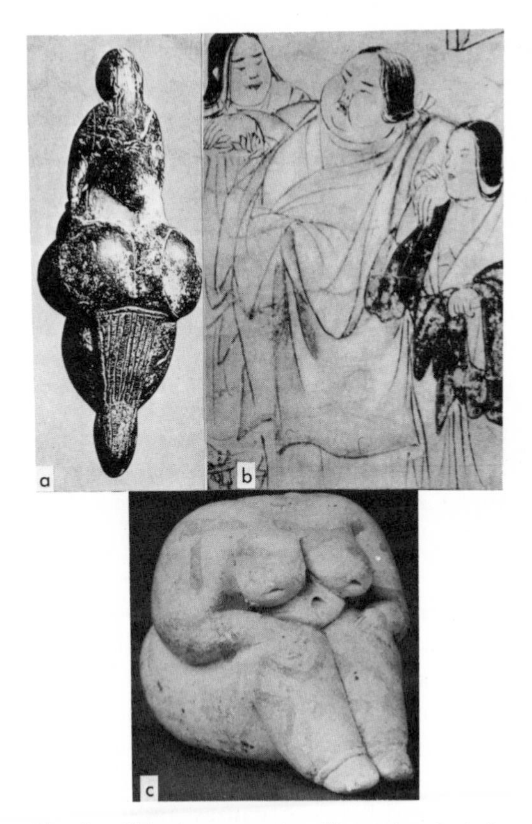

Fig. 3. Old statuettes and an illustration depicting obese subjects. a: Venus of Lespugue from behind (made of mammoth ivory in France; 25,000-21,000 B.C.). b: from Yamai-zoshi (a rolled book illustrating many morbid states made in Japan more than 800 years ago). c: statuette of a seated goddess (baked clay belonging to Anatolian civilization; 5,500 B.C.).

heavy, but this does not necessarily mean that all of them have marked fat accumulation. Bodies of some of these wrestlers show extremely high muscularity. The CT scan imaging at the level of the umbilicus of the usual young sumo wrestler is something like Fig. 4. It clearly shows the presence of markedly high muscularity, (as compared with Fig. 1), which is associated with subcutaneous fat accumulation; the visceral fat is rather scanty. The incidence of

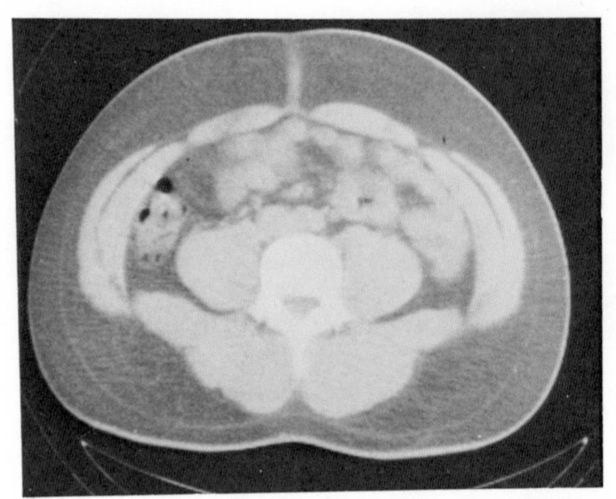

Fig. 4. Representative CT scan imaging at the level of the umbilicus of a young Sumo wrestler (body mass index: 32).

glucose intolerance among active sumo wrestlers has been said to be elevated, but in fact it is not so high, taking the marked degree of overweight and overeating into consideration. Many active sumo wrestlers still maintain normal glucose tolerance and normal lipidemia. However, the incidence of glycosuria is about 30% among retired sumo wrestlers who have ceased the habit of muscle training.

Three possibilities seem likely as causes inducing visceral obesity, particularly in modern, advanced societies: overeating of refined sugars, overeating of high fat diet and decreased energy turnover through reduced muscular exercise. Our preliminary animal experiments suggest that at least the overeating of refined sugars could cause an accumulation of mesenteric fat.

V. REVERSIBILITY OF INTRAABDOMINAL FAT ACCUMULATION

The last important question is: can the restriction of calorie intake and increased muscular exercise reduce the visceral fat? The answer is "yes" from our recent observations. Figure 5 is a representative case of a 35-year old female. The intraabdominal fat

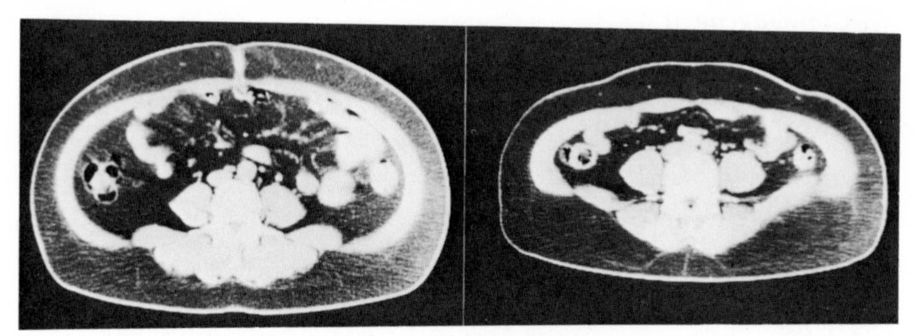

Fig. 5. Alteration of visceral fat through diet and exercise therapy. Before therapy (left) and 4 months after beginning therapy (right).

accumulation was markedly reduced after diet and exercise therapy for four months. In general, percentage of visceral fat in total body fat was significantly decreased after therapy in groups with visceral type obesity. Visceral fat thus seems to be rather sensitive to calorie restriction and exercise therapy.

When V/S ratio was reduced more than 0.1 after the diet and exercise therapy, significant improvements in metabolic parameters, including plasma glucose area on OGTT, total cholesterol and triglyceride were observed. The more marked the decrease in V/S ratio was, the more significant was the improvement demonstrated in metabolic derangement.

SUMMARY

Human obesity is a heterogeneous condition from the aspect of topographical fat distribution. Our analyses using CT scan imaging indicated that human obesity could be classified into two categories: subcutaneous-type and visceral-type. Disturbances in glucose and lipid metabolism are more marked in the visceral-type than in the subcutaneous-type. However, visceral fat is rather sensitive to calorie restriction and exercise therapy, and can be reduced through the efforts of a subject with visceral-type obesity.

Acknowledgement

We would like to express our sincere gratitude for the advice about the "Gilgamesh" epic provided by Prof. Mamoru Yoshikawa of Hiroshima University.

REFERENCES

1. Kissebah, A.H., Vydelingum, H., and Murray, R. (1982). Relation of body fat distribution to metabolic complications of obesity. *J. Clin. Endocrinol. Metab.* **54**, 254-260.
2. Krotkiewski, M., Bjorntorp, P., and Sjostrom, L. (1983). Impact of obesity on metabolism in men and women—importance of regional adipose tissue distribution. *J. Clin. Invest.* **72**, 1150-1162.
3. Vague, J. (1947). La differenciation sexuelle—facteur determinant des formes de l'obesitĉ. *Presse Med.* **30**, 339-340.
4. Fujioka, S., Matsuzawa, Y., Tokunaga, K., and Tarui, S. (1987). Contribution of intra-abdominal fat accumulation to the impairment of glucose and lipid metabolism in human obesity. *Metabolism* **36**, 54-59.
5. Tokunaga, K., Matsuzawa, Y., Ishikawa, K., and Tarui, S. (1983). A novel technique for the determination of body fat by computed tomography. *Int. J. Obesity* **7**, 437-445.
6. Tippett, P.S. and Kenneth, E.N. (1982). Specific inhibition of glucokinase by long chain acyl coenzymes A below the critical micelle concentration. *J. Biol. Chem.* **257**, 12839-12845.
7. Ramadoss, C.S., Uyeda, K., and Johnston, J.M. (1976). Studies on the fatty acid inactivation of phosphofructokinase. *J. Biol. Chem.* **251**, 98-107.
8. Garland, P.B., Randle, P.J., and Newsholme, E.A. (1963). Citrate as an intermediary in the inhibition of phosphofructokinase in rat heart muscle by fatty acids, ketone bodies, pyruvate, diabetes and starvation. *Nature* **200**, 169-170.
9. Hue, L., Maisin, L., and Rider, M.H. (1988). Palmitate inhibits liver glycolysis. *Biochem. J.* **251**, 541-545.

Diet and Obesity, Bray, G.A. et al., eds., pp. 153-161.
Japan Sci. Soc. Press, Tokyo/S. Karger, Basel (1988)

Sweet Foods and Sweeteners in the U.S. Diet

ADAM DREWNOWSKI

Human Nutrition Program, School of Public Health and Department of Psychiatry, Medical School, The University of Michigan, Ann Arbor, MI 48109, U.S.A.

Approximately 32 million American adults between 25 and 74 years of age are reported to be overweight. This figure represents 28% of the entire adult population of the United States (*1*). These estimates are derived from the National Health and Nutrition Examinations Survey (NHANES II 1976-1980), which includes health histories, physical exam data, and dietary interviews for over 20,000 persons between 3 and 74 years of age. Conducted by the National Center for Health Statistics, this survey monitors the relationship between nutrient composition of the diet and obesity, diabetes, hypertension, and heart disease. The risks of having diabetes, hypertension, and elevated serum lipid levels are commonly higher among persons who are overweight than among those who are not (*2, 3*).

Several studies have linked the increasing prevalence of obesity and its associated diseases with the increasing sugar and fat content of the American diet (*3*). The average adult consumes between 60 and 90 g of fat and an estimated 95 g of sugar per day. The health aspects of sugars contained in carbohydrate sweeteners have received particularly close attention (*4*), and there is a need for accurate estimates of sugar consumption in the U.S. diet. The available estimates of consumption of sugar and other sweeteners are generally based on two types of measures: food disappearance statistics and the analysis of food intake records.

I. HISTORICAL TRENDS

Data collected by the U.S. Department of Agriculture are often expressed as "disappearance" statistics. These are based on supply data for 350 foods as they disappear into the foods supply, rather than on how much is eaten. These data are adjusted for exports and stockpiling, but are not adjusted for food waste, further processing or animal use. Actual consumption is thought to be between 10 and 30% less than indicated by the disappearance figures.

Food disappearance data collected since the beginning of the century provide an index of historical trends in the U.S. food supply. It is well known that the amount of available fats has risen by 30% since 1910, while available carbohydrates have declined by

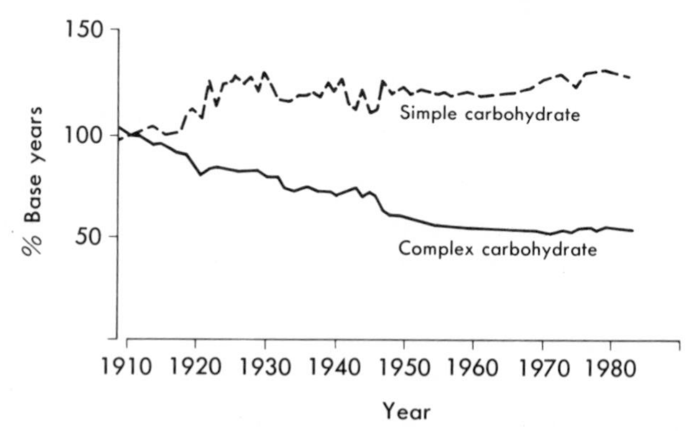

Fig. 1. Carbohydrates in the U.S. food supply. Simple and complex carbohydrates as percent of base years: 1909–1913 = 154 g simple carbohydrate and 336 g complex carbohydrate/capita/day. Sources: data from the U.S. food supply historical series and 1955, 1965, and 1977–1978 food consumption surveys.

more than 20%. However, as shown in Fig. 1, the steady decline in the use of complex carbohydrates (primarily potatoes and grain products) has been offset by increased use of sugars and other caloric sweeteners. Per capita consumption of caloric sweeteners reached a high of 142.5 pounds a year in 1984 (that is an average of 600 sweet calories per day), compared to 65 pounds in 1900. Recent statistics indicate that sugars contribute 17% of calories to the U.S. diet.

The composition of dietary sweeteners has also changed. The consumption of cane and beet sugar (sucrose) has been declining during the past decade, down to 67.5 pounds per person in 1984. This decline was caused by the increased use of corn-derived sweeteners, particularly high-fructose corn syrup (HFCS), and the expanding application of artificial sweeteners. Between 1967–1969 and 1983, the use of corn syrup climbed from 16 to 65.6 pounds per person, while the total use of HFCS rose from 1 pound per person in 1970 to 43.2 lbs in 1983 (*5*). Most recent statistics place the current use of corn sweeteners at 74.7 pounds per person, above the current consumption of sucrose.

The changing nature of the soft drinks industry has been responsible for some of these trends. Industry figures show that soft drink sales have more than doubled from 1970 to 1985 from an equivalent of 49.5 billion of 12-ounce cans to 116.1 billion. Per capita consumption rose from 9.6 ounces per day to 16 ounces per day in 1985. However, the use of sucrose in soft drinks dropped from 25 lbs per capita in 1980 to 8 lbs per capita in 1984, when it was replaced by the cheaper HFCS as the single caloric sweetener in both Coca-Cola and Pepsi-Cola. HFCS use in soft drinks accounted for over two-thirds of the estimated 4.3 million tons of total HFCS consumption in 1984.

The current popularity of non-caloric soft drinks reflects increased public concern with health and dieting. Diet soft drinks represented 23.1% of the soft drink market, up from 10% in 1975. The total consumption of saccharin was estimated at 10 pounds per person in 1984, while the consumption of aspartame (Nutrasweet) was 5.8 pounds per person and growing.

II. MEASURES OF SUGAR INTAKE

What are the chief sources of sugar in the American diet? How much sugar do individuals actually consume? Some of these questions can be answered by examining individual records of food intake for large population samples, stratified by both sex and age.

The Nationwide Food Consumption Survey (NFCS) examines household food use and individual food intakes. Last conducted in 1977–1978 by the U.S. Department of Agriculture, the NFCS examined 15,000 households using a 7-day record of foods used. Individual respondents recalled one days' food intake and kept a diary for 2 additional days. According to survey estimates, protein currently accounts for 17%, fat for 41%, and carbohydrate for 43% of food calories in the U.S. diet (*6*). The major sources of energy are meat, poultry, fish and grain products (*6* , *7*).

The summary of sugars intake is provided in Table I. The sugars are divided into those naturally present in foods (in milk, fruits or honey) and those added during the manufacturing process to processed foods. The data are presented as both grams per day and as percent of calories in the average American diet.

Mean daily intake of sugars is known to vary for different

TABLE I
Sweeteners in the U.S. Diet: Summary of Sugars Intake (NFCS 1977–1978)

	Intake (g/day)	Percent of calories
Sucrose		
Added	28	6
Natural	13	3
Fructose		
Added	10	2
Natural	7	2
Corn sweeteners		
HFCS	19	4
Others	6	1
Total	81	18

TABLE II
Sugars in the U.S. Diet: Average Daily Intake of Sugars, Carbohydrate and Calories (NFCS 1977-1978)

	Grams per day			CHO (g)	Calories per day
	Added sugars	Natural sugars	Total sugars		
Males					
11-14 yrs	76	57	123	257	2252
15-18 yrs	84	59	143	283	2578
19-22 yrs	73	47	121	248	2403
23-50 yrs	62	43	105	230	2330
>50 yrs	48	45	92	206	2042
Females					
11-14 yrs	65	47	112	214	1856
15-18 yrs	62	41	103	196	1746
19-22 yrs	52	34	86	170	1600
23-50 yrs	44	33	74	158	1548
>50 yrs	35	38	74	155	1470

population groups. The reported daily intakes of sugars, carbohydrate and calories are presented in Table II. The daily intake of added sugars for the different population subgroups ranged between 10 and 84 g per day, with a mean of 53 g per day for the total population. The intake of naturally occurring sugars (mostly lactose from milk) ranged from 33 to 59 g per day (mean: 42 g per day), while the values for total sugars ranged from 62 to 143 g per day, with a mean of 95 g per day for the total population (*4*).

The same data, expressed as percent total daily calories are shown in Table III. It can be seen that the highest percentage of total calories derived from sugar (22-24%) is observed for the two youngest age groups: children and teenagers. There has been some concern that these groups are most susceptible to the adverse health effects of excessive sugar consumption (*4*). Studies on the development of food preferences suggest that young children best like familiar sweet foods. In sensory evaluation studies, children often fail to show the customary breakpoint for sucrose, preferring instead the most intense sucrose concentrations. Several investigators have suggested that the high sugar content of foods frequently consumed

TABLE III
Sugars in the U.S. Diet: Average Daily Intake of Sugars and Carbohydrate as Percent of Calories (USDA NFCS 1977–1978)

	Added sugars	Natural sugars	Total sugars	Carbohydrate
Males				
11–14 yrs	13	10	23	46
15–18 yrs	13	9	22	44
19–22 yrs	12	8	20	42
23–50 yrs	11	7	18	39
>50 yrs	9	9	18	41
Females				
11–14 yrs	14	10	24	46
15–18 yrs	14	9	24	45
19–22 yrs	13	9	22	43
23–50 yrs	11	9	20	41
>50 yrs	9	11	20	42

by children and adolescents is directly linked to the development of childhood and juvenile onset obesity.

The nutrient composition of foods reported to be highly preferred by children deserves further examination. The Nutrient Data Bank provides a list of over 60 nutrients for a large portion of some 10,000–15,000 foods in the U.S. food supply. This list is updated on a continuing basis by the USDA Nutrient Composition Lab (Beltsville, MD), and is the source for the USDA Handbook No. 8. Other nutrient databases include the Michigan State University Nutrient Data Bank, which lists sugar content for a large number of brand name foods, including sweets, candy, and other desserts.

Analyses of NHANES II data (*7*) show that the chief sources of dietary carbohydrate in the U.S. diet include bread, soft drinks, doughnuts, cookies, milk, fried potatoes, alcohol, and orange juice. Many of these products contain added sugar: soft drinks, pastries, and sugar together contribute almost 20% of the total carbohydrate intake. Among other products containing appreciable amounts of added sugar are milk beverages, yogurts, ice cream, puddings and

TABLE IV
Nutrient Composition of Foods: Chocolate Candy (per package or bar)

	Total (kcal)	Sugar (kcal)	Fat (kcal)	S+F/T (%)
M&M/Mars Plain Chocolate Candies	237	109	123	98
M&M/Mars Peanut Chocolate Candies	241	88	108	81
M&M/Mars Snickers Bar	274	116	117	85
M&M/Mars Milky Way Bar	268	144	90	87
Hershey Milk Chocolate with Almonds Bar	226	80	126	91
Hershey Special Dark Chocolate Candy	222	80	108	85
Nestle Crunch Bar	156	60	72	85

TABLE V
Nutrient Composition of Foods: Cookies (per cookie)

	Total (kcal)	Sugar (kcal)	Fat (kcal)	S+F/T (%)
Nabisco Chips Ahoy	52	12	18	58
Nabisco Oreo Cookies	52	16	18	66
Nabisco Fudge Cream Sandwich	52	16	18	66
Nabisco Peanut-Cream Patties	110	24	54	71
Pepperidge Farm Geneva	63	16	36	82
Pepperidge Farm Chocolate Chip	50	16	18	68
Pepperidge Farm Date-Nut Granola Cookies	107	24	51	70

other milk desserts, muffins, biscuits, doughnuts, cake, cookies, pies, cereals, syrups, dessert toppings, jams, preserves, gelatin desserts, popsicles, all candies, and chewing gums (*4, 7*).

However, sugar in many "sweet" foods may not be the chief source of energy. Analysis of the sugar and fat content of selected candies, cookies, and desserts shows that sugar and fat together may account for up to 98% of total calories. Fat calories often exceed sugar calories, as demonstrated in Tables IV and V.

TABLE VI
Sugars in the U.S. Diet: Mean Daily Sugar Intake (g) by Children Ages 5–12 ($n=657$) Based on 7-Day Diaries

Food group	Mean (g)	Percent of total sugar
Breakfast cereals	4.2	3.3
Cakes, cookies, pies	15.3	11.2
Candy	3.7	2.6
Breads, doughnuts, rolls	7.4	5.7
Fruit	17.1	11.5
Fruit juices	12.0	8.8
Jellies, sauces, syrups, and table sugar	17.3	12.3
Milk	25.9	20.4
Sweetened beverages	17.9	13.8
Sweet dairy products	7.4	5.5
Other foods	6.1	4.9
All foods (total)	134.3	100.0

Morgan and Zabik (*8*)

The intake of foods containing mixtures of sugar and fat should be monitored most closely. Previous analyses have been concerned with the consumption of sugar alone. For example, presweetened cereals and candy have been mentioned as the chief sources of sugar for children. However, studies based on NFCS Survey show that fully 20% of sugars consumed by children ages 5–12 are derived from natural milk (lactose), followed by sweetened soft drinks (14%). As shown in Table VI, candy and sweet dairy products (ice cream) contribute a much lower proportion of sugar calories; their contribution to fat consumption, however, may be considerable.

SUMMARY

The current status of sugars in the U.S. diet is characterized by the declining use of sucrose and its replacement by corn sweeteners, particularly HFCS. The two sugars have different insulinogenic properties, and their impact on the development of childhood or juvenile onset obesity remains to be evaluated. Changing attitudes towards weight and dieting may also result in shifting patterns of sugar intake. Consumer surveys show that more than 68 million Americans, age 18 and over, use low-calorie foods and beverages. This represents an increase of more than 60% since 1978. The long-term impact of non-caloric sweeteners in soft drinks and other food products is also a target for further studies in nutritional epidemiology.

REFERENCES

1. Abraham, S. and Johnson, C.L. (1980). Prevalence of severe obesity in adults in the United States. *Am. J. Clin. Nutr.* **33**, 364–369.
2. National Institutes of Health (1985). Health implications of obesity. NIH Consensus Development Conference. National Institutes of Health, Bethesda, MD.
3. Van Itallie, T.B. (1979). Obesity: adverse effects on health and longevity. *Am. J. Clin. Nutr.* **32**, 2723–2733.
4. Glinsman, W.H., Irausquin, H., and Park, Y.K. (1986). Evaluation of health aspects of sugars contained in carbohydrate sweeteners: Report of the Sugars Task Force. *J. Nutr.* **116**(11S), S1–216.
5. Marston, R.M. and Raper, N.R. (1985). The nutrient content of the food supply. *Natl. Food Rev.* **29**, 5–7.
6. U.S. Department of Health and Human Services and U.S. Department of Agriculture (1986) Nutrition Monitoring in the United States. DHHS Publ. No. (PHS) 86-1255. Public Health Service., U.S. Government Printing Office, Washington, D.C.
7. Block, G., Dresser, C.M., Hartman, A.M., and Carroll, M.D. (1985). Nutrient sources in the American diet: Quantitative data from the NHANES II survey. *Am. J. Epidemiol.* **122**, 27–40.
8. Morgan, K.J. and Zabik, M.E. (1981). Amount and food sources of total sugar intake by children ages 5 to 12 years. *Am. J. Clin. Nutr.* **34**, 404–413.

Diet and Obesity, Bray, G.A. et al., eds., pp. 163–173.
Japan Sci. Soc. Press, Tokyo/S. Karger, Basel (1988)

Sweeteners: Low-energetic and Low-insulinogenic

MASASHIGE SUZUKI AND TOMOHIRO TAMURA

Biochemistry of Exercise and Nutrition, Institute of Health and Sport Sciences, The University of Tsukuba, Tsukuba 305, Japan

The average daily intake of sucrose in 1980 was about 58 g per person in Japan (9% of daily energy intake of 2,590 kcal), 110 g in Canada (14% of 3,140 kcal), and 150 g in the U.S. (18% of 3,390 kcal) (Table I) (*1*). The sucrose intake in Japan increased continuously until 1979 but decreased slightly thereafter, while corn sweeteners have rapidly increased during the last decade (Fig. 1) (*1*). Recently, there has been a progressive increase in the use of new sweeteners such as sugar alcohols (sorbitol, maltitol, *etc.*), sweeteners derived from sucrose (palatinose, fructoligosaccharide, coupling sugar, *etc.*), non-carbohydrate sugars (stevia, *etc.*) and artificial sweeteners (aspartame, *etc.*) (Fig. 2) (*2*).

I. SWEETENERS: CALORIGENICITY AND INSULINOGENICITY

These sweeteners can be divided into three major groups by their nutritional effects such as calorigenicity and insulinogenicity: insulinogenic-calorigenic, low-insulinogenic-calorigenic, and low-insulinogenic-low calorigenic. Not only the calorigenicity but also

TABLE I
Daily Energy Intake from Sugars by the Japanese, Canadians, and Americans (*1*)

	Total calorie (kcal)	Starch (g)	Sugars (g)	Fat (g)	Protein (g)
Japanese[a]	2,590	310	58(9)*	79	81
Canadians[b]	3,140	204	110(14)	151	98
Americans[c]	3,390	186	153(18)	166	106

[a]1982; [b,c]1987. ( )*, % of total calories.

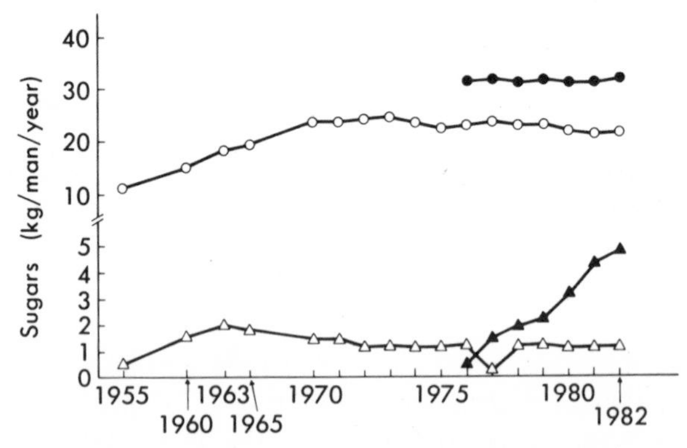

Fig. 1. Changes in annual consumption of sucrose, corn-sweeteners and glucose by Japanese (*2*). ● total; ○ sucrose; ▲ corn-sweetener.

the insulinogenicity of the sweeteners is involved in the accumulation of excess body fat, because insulin stimulates the activity of adipose tissue lipoprotein lipase which is the key enzyme regulating the uptake and storage of blood triglycerides as body fat.

II. BODY FAT ACCUMULATION AND ACTIVATION OF LIPOPROTEIN LIPASE IN ADIPOSE TISSUE BY INSULINOGENIC SUGARS

It seems very important to note that this increase in sugar consumption has generally occurred with modernization, in parallel with the increase in fat consumption seen in Japan (Fig. 3) (*3*). The reason this should be looked at is that we have demonstrated in rats

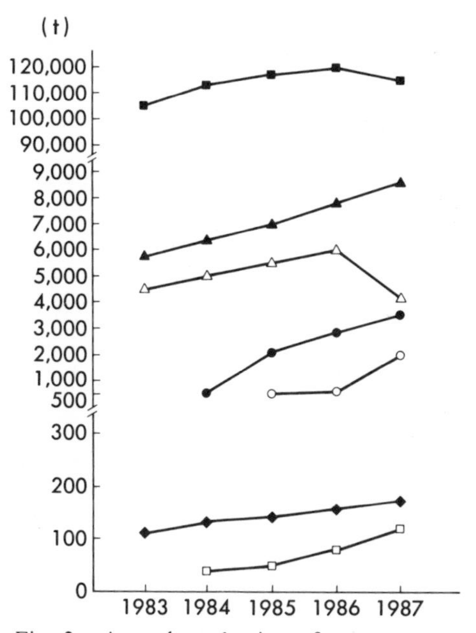

Fig. 2. Annual production of new sweeteners in Japan (*2*). ■ sorbitol; ▲ maltitol; △ coupling sugar; ○ palatinose; ◆ stevia; □ aspartame.

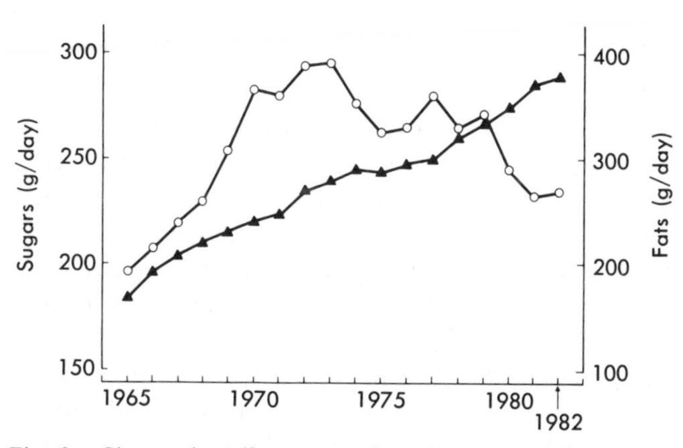

Fig. 3. Changes in daily consumption of sugars and fat by Japanese (*3*). ○ sugars; ▲ fats.

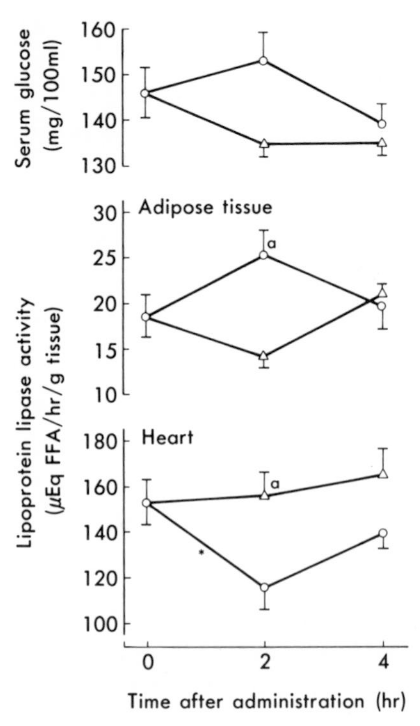

Fig. 4. Responses of lipoprotein lipase activity in adipose tissue and heart to the oral administration of glucose or maltitol in rats (*5*). ○ glucose; △ maltitol. [a]$p<0.05$, *$p<0.05$.

that the accumulation of excess body fat is apparently related to the consumption of a high fat diet together with an insulinogenic sugar such as sucrose (*4*). This mechanism is explained as one in which the ingestion of insulinogenic sugar, sucrose, together with fat opens the fat gate of the adipose tissue by stimulating its lipoprotein lipase while chylomicron triglycerides are secreted into the blood in large quantities.

Our data suggest that the increased prevalence of eating fatty foods together with insulinogenic sugars in the modernization of food habits might be strongly related to the increased rate of obesity generally seen in industrialized countries. Therefore, an important

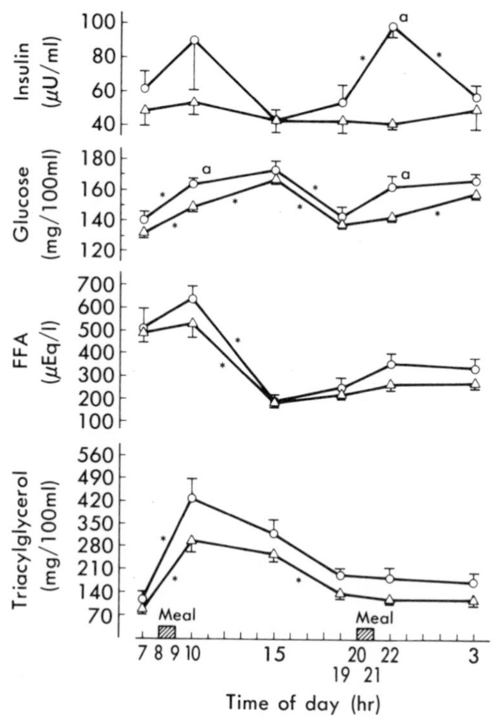

Fig. 5. Diurnal changes in serum concentrations of insulin, glucose, free fatty acid and triacylglycerol in rats meal-fed on a maltitol- or sucrose-added high fat diet (*5*). ○ sucrose; △ maltitol. $^{a}p<0.05$, $^{*}p<0.05$.

dietary effort in the prevention of excessive body fat accumulation is either to avoid the simultaneous ingestion of fatty foods and insulinogenic sugars or to use low-insulinogenic sugars for the preparation of fatty-sweet foods.

III. EFFECTIVE PREVENTION OF EXCESSIVE BODY FAT ACCUMULATION BY LOW-INSULINOGENIC SWEETENER IN HIGH FAT MEAL

We compared the body fat accumulation between a sucrose-added high fat meal and a low-insulinogenic sugar, maltitol-added

TABLE II
Dietary Composition (*5*)

	Diets	
	Fat-sucrose (g)	Fat-maltitol (g)
CE-2	54	54
Casein	10	10
Soybean oil	17	17
Sucrose	15	—
Maltitol	—	15
Minerals	3.5	3.5
Vitamins	0.5	0.5
	(% of total calories)	
Carbohydrate	39.0	
(Sugar)	(13.7)	
Fat	39.7	
Protein	21.3	

high fat meal in rats (*5*). Maltitol, α-1,4-glucosyl-sorbitol, is a sweetener produced by hydrogenation of maltose. Maltitol is not digestible in the stomach and small intestine but is fermented almost completely by microflora into volatile fatty acids and other acids in the large intestine (*6*). Therefore, the caloric value of maltitol is estimated to be almost equal to that of sucrose (*7*).

When 30 g of maltitol was orally given to a fasted human, there were only slight responses in serum glucose, insulin or RQ values, in contrast with sharp increases in these parameters after sucrose administration (Fig. 4). Although insulinogenic sugars such as sucrose and glucose inhibit or stimulate lipoprotein lipase activity in the cardiac and muscle tissues or the adipose tissue, respectively, maltitol does not influence activity of these tissue lipoprotein lipases at all (Fig. 5). If we consider these different nutritional characteristics between sucrose and maltitol, it could be speculated that, as compared with a sucrose-added high fat meal, a maltitol-added high fat meal could give lower blood glucose level and insulin secretion, which would lead to lower adipose tissue lipoprotein lipase activity and result in lower body fat accumulation.

TABLE III
Effect of a 6-Month Feeding of a Maltitol- or Sucrose-added High Fat Diet on Weight Gain and Organ and Tissue Weights in Rats (*5*)

	Dietary		Significance
	Fat-sucrose (*27*)	Fat-maltitol (*30*)	
Body weight (g)			
Initial	217±1	217±1	$p<0.01$
Final	624±4	602±6	$p<0.01$
Gain	407±4	385±6	
Liver (g)	16.1±0.2	16.0±0.2	
Lungs (g)	1.9±0.1	1.9±0.1	
Heart (g)	1.3±0.0	1.3±0.0	
Spleen (g)	0.8±0.0	0.8±0.0	
Kidneys (g)	3.0±0.1	2.9±0.0	
Soleus muscle (g)	0.4±0.0	0.4±0.0	
Adipose tissue (g)			
Epididymal	18.9±0.7	16.7±0.5	$p<0.05$
Perirenal	30.2±1.3	25.4±1.1	$p<0.01$
Mesenteric	17.7±0.9	14.4±0.7	$p<0.01$
Total	66.7±2.5	56.8±2.1	$p<0.01$
Stomach (g)	2.6±0.1	2.4±0.1	$p<0.05$
Small intestime (g)	8.1±0.4	9.4±0.5	$p<0.05$
Caecum (g)	1.6±0.1	1.9±0.1	$p<0.001$
Large intestine (g)	2.4±0.1	3.2±0.1	$p<0.001$

Mean±SEM. ( ), number of rats.

Therefore, two experimental diets were prepared by adding sucrose or maltitol 15% by weight to a semipurified high fat diet; 40% of the total energy of the diets was provided by fat, 39% by carbohydrate and 13.7% sucrose or maltitol (Table II). Male Sprague-Dawley rats 6 weeks of age were meal-fed twice a day. Two dietary groups were fed the same amount at each meal. Both groups initially showed a similar weight gain, but the maltitol group later showed a smaller weight gain and had significantly lower body weight at the end of the feeding period (Table III). The rats were killed at 6 time-points on the final day of the experiment. Both groups showed the same sizes in various organs and skeletal muscle, but the weight of the intra-abdominal adipose tissue in the maltitol

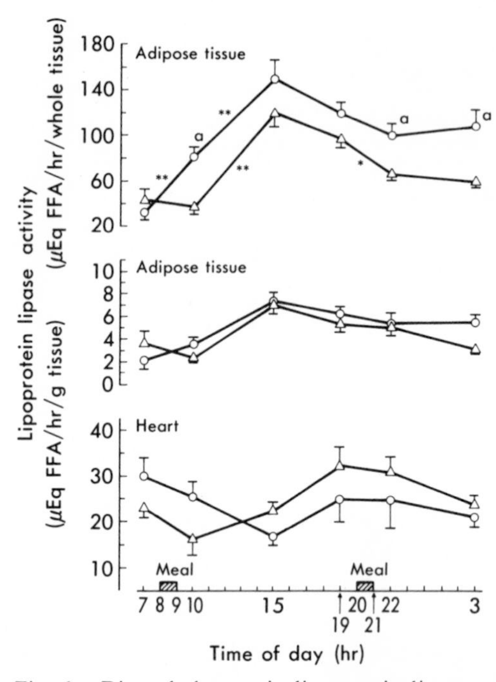

Fig. 6. Diurnal changes in lipoprotein lipase activity in adipose tissue and heart in rats meal-fed on a maltitol- or sucrose-added high fat diet (*5*). ○ sucrose; △ maltitol. [a]$p<0.05$, *$p<0.05$, **$p<0.01$.

group was significantly lower in all animals. A significant hypertrophy of the digestive tract occurred in this group, and animals showed significantly lower serum levels in glucose, insulin and triglyceride than the sucrose group did (Fig. 6). Adipose tissue lipoprotein lipase activity expressed not on a tissue paragram but on a whole tissue basis was significantly lower in the maltitol group than the sucrose group (Fig. 7). The analyses of body composition were very interesting: although protein content was the same between the groups, fat content was significantly less in the maltitol group (Table IV).

The results demonstrate that substitution of insulinogenic sucrose by low-insulinogenic maltitol is effective in preventing exces-

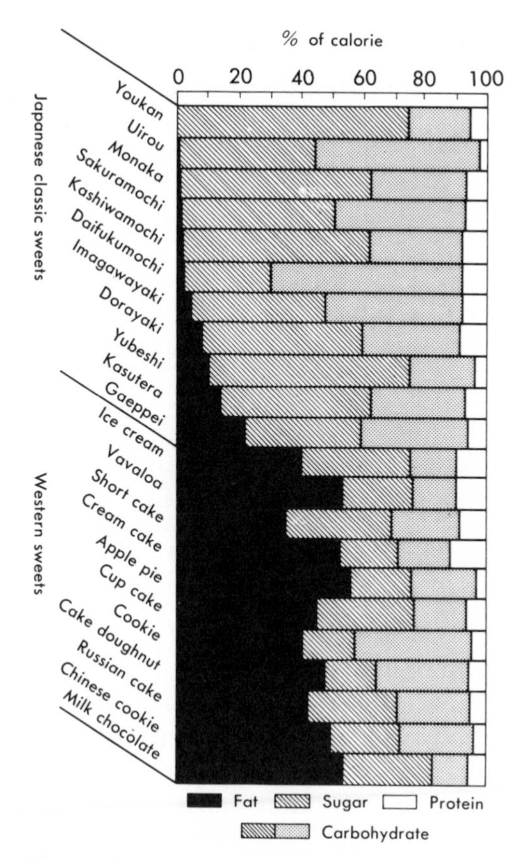

Fig. 7. Fat and sugar composition of Japanese and Western sweets (*8*).

sive body fat accumulation caused by the simultaneous ingestion of fat and sucrose. Thus, our results suggest that low-insulinogenic sugars have an important role in the prevention of the accumulation of excess body fat in organisms which habitually consume high fat meals.

Furthermore, it could be suggested to the sweet-food producers that low-insulinogenic sweeteners are possibly not effective for insulinogenic starchy-foods such as classic Japanese sweets, in which low-calorie sweeteners may be much more valuable. On the other

TABLE IV
Effect of a 6-Month Feeding of a Maltitol- or Sucrose-added High Fat Diet on Weight and Body Protein and Fat Content in Rats (*5*)

	Dietary		Significance
	Fat-sucrose (*27*)	Fat-maltitol (*29*)	
Carcass weight (g)	418±3	396±4	$p<0.001$
Carcass+adipose tissue			
Weight	475±5	446±5	$p<0.001$
Protein (g)	79±1	79±1	
(%)	19±0	20±0	$p<0.05$
Fat (g)	142±6	113±5	$p<0.001$
(%)	30±1	25±1	$p<0.001$

Mean±SEM. ( ), number of rats.

hand, the low-caloric sweeteners may not be as physiologically beneficial in high calorie fatty-foods such as Western sweets (Fig. 7) (*8*).

SUMMARY

Substitution of insulinogenic sucrose by a low-insulinogenic sugar, maltitol, was effective in preventing excessive body fat accumulation by feeding a sucrose-added high fat meal in rats. This suggests that low-insulinogenic sugars have an important role in the prevention of obesity in humans in industrialized countries where fatty foods are habitually consumed. Effectiveness of utilization of low-calorigenic or low-insulinogenic sweeteners for fatty-foods and starchy-foods was briefly discussed.

REFERENCES

1. Report on "Sucrose and Health," by Working Group for Sucrose, ILSI Japan, Tokyo, pp. 1–11 (1985).
2. Report on "Sweeteners Market," by Kaken Marketing, Tokyo, pp. 1–188 (1987).
3. Japanese Ministry of Agriculture Forestry and Fisheries, Tables of Food Consumption and Production (1986).
4. Suzuki, S. and Tamura, T. This volume, pp. 113–119.
5. Suzuki, S. and Tamura, T. (1987). A smaller body fat accumulation by the feeding

of a high fat diet together with a non-insulinogenic sugar, maltitol, than sucrose in rats. *Fed. Proc.* **46**, 881.
6. Dahlqvist, A. and Telenius, U. (1965). The utilization of a presumably low-calorigenic carbohydrate derivative. *Acta Physiol. Scand.* **63**, 156–163.
7. Rennhard, H.H. and Bianchine, J.R. (1976). Metabolism and caloric utilization of orally administrated maltitol-^{14}C in rat. *J. Agric. Food Chem.* **24**, 287–291.
8. Japanese Agency of Science and Technology, Investigation Committee of National Resources (1983). Standard tables of food composition in Japan, 4th ed.

Diet and Obesity, Bray, G.A. et al., eds., pp. 175–180.
Japan Sci. Soc. Press, Tokyo/S. Karger, Basel (1988)

Adipose Tissue Cellularity and Function and Food Intake Regulation

JUDITH S. STERN

Department of Nutrition, Food Intake Laboratory and Division of Clinical Nutrition in the Department of Internal Medicine, University of California, Davis, California 95616, U.S.A.

Obesity is defined as an increase in the mass of adipose tissue. This may be accomplished by an increase in fat cell size or fat cell number or an increase in both fat cell size and number. Once obesity is established, weight reduction is accomplished by a decrease in fat cell size; fat cell number is relatively unchanged.

There is increasing evidence that regional differences in adipose tissue morphology and metabolism may be associated with altered risk for chronic diseases such as diabetes, hypertension, and cardiovascular disease. While this research is ongoing and it is difficult, at this time, to precisely identify mechanisms, it does emphasize the importance of studying adipose tissue cellularity, fat distribution, and metabolism in obesity.

I. CELLULARITY AND FUNCTION

Studies by Jules Hirsch and his colleagues have been seminal to studies of adipose cellularity. They demonstrated that preweaning over- and underfeeding affect the ultimate number of fat cells found in the epididymal depot of the adult rat. Knittle and Hirsch raised rats in large litters (22 pups per litter) to limit food intake and in small litters (4 pups per litter) to maximize the quantity of milk available (*1*). At 3 weeks of age, rats were weaned and allowed to eat a stock diet *ad libitum* for an additional 17 weeks. Both adipose cell size and number in the epididymal depots were still increased at 20 weeks of age. Similar studies in the genetically obese Zucker rat (*fa/fa*) extended these findings (*2*). While overfeeding genetically obese rats during the preweaning period increased adult fat cell number, underfeeding did not result in a lower fat cell number in comparison to *ad libitum* fed obese controls.

Subsequent studies have revealed that while overfeeding the rat during the preweaning period can markedly alter adult fat cell number and size, adult rats that are fed a high fat diet also increase fat cell number and size. In one study, 9 weeks of high fat feeding commencing at 13 weeks of age resulted in a doubling of fat cell number and an increase in fat cell size in the retroperitoneal depot of male Osborne-Mendel rats (*3*). When these rats were refed a stock diet (Purina chow) for an additional 20 weeks, fat cell size returned to normal but fat cell number was still elevated. Thus, rats fed a high fat diet for only 2 months followed by almost 5 months of low fat feeding have elevated body fat. In this same study, high sucrose feeding for 5 months also resulted in increases in fat cell number in adult rats (*3*).

This increase in adipose cellularity in response to a palatable diet is not limited to young adults. In a subsequent study, we demonstrated that an increase in fat cell number also occurred when 22 month-old female Sprague-Dawley rats were fed a high fat diet for only one week (*4*). We reported an increase in ^{3}H-thymidine incorporation into DNA isolated from retroperitoneal adipocytes. This was confirmed by radioautography.

Whether adult humans also increase fat cell number in response to a palatable diet is not known. However, since long term success in treating obesity is limited, it seems appropriate to limit the quantity of food as well as the fat and sucrose content of the diet.

There are a number of studies that support the observation that those formerly obese individuals who maintain a reduced body weight appear to incorporate exercise into their daily routine (*5*). Data from experimental animals are supportive of this observation.

Lipoprotein lipase (LPL) is a key enzyme for the storage of circulating triglycerides in adipose tissue. In the genetically obese Zucker rat, exercise is associated with decreased LPL activity in adipose tissue and increased LPL activity in muscle (*6*). Within a few days of cessation of exercise, adipose tissue LPL activity is elevated (*7*). This is consistent with an increase in food intake, plasma insulin levels, and rapid regain of body weight and fat. Recent data from our laboratory has also demonstrated that the cessation of exercise is associated with an increase in fat cell number as measured by an increase of ^{3}H-thymidine incorporation into fat cell DNA (*8*).

II. FAT DISTRIBUTION

There is increasing evidence that adipose tissue is not uniform and that there are regional differences in its morphology, metabolism, and responses to certain hormones. LPL activity, key for the storage of circulating triglycerides in adipose tissue, can vary in the abdominal and femoral regions as a function of sex and reproductive status. Males have increased LPL activity in the abdominal region in comparison to the femoral region (*9*). This is consistent with an upper body fat distribution commonly found in males. LPL activity is higher in the femoral region that in the abdominal region in premenopausal women (*10*). Pregnancy, a time of rapid fat deposition, further elevated LPL activity in the femoral region (*11*). This is consistent with a lower body fat distribution commonly seen in women. Lactation, a time of fat mobilization, is associated with a drop in LPL activity in the femoral region (*11*). With menopause, LPL activity decreases in both abdominal and femoral regions (*9, 10*). It is not clear, from studies in humans, which of the female sex hormones is the most important for LPL activity in the femoral region. In rats, progesterone appears to be vital, however, estrogen is needed for progesterone to be effective (*12, 13*).

These regional differences could have significant impact on some of the health risks associated with obesity. It has been proposed that fat distribution can predict some of the metabolic abnormalities seen in obesity. In one study, plasma glucose and insulin levels were significantly higher in women with upper body obesity than in women with lower body obesity (*14*). In this study, upper body obesity was associated with hypertrophy of fat cells, whereas lower body obesity was associated with normal cell size.

III. FOOD INTAKE

Adipose tissue derived signals which could drive feeding behavior have been sought for a number of decades. Several candidates, including steroidal products, glycerol, and free fatty acids have all proved to be important but not uniquely stimulatory of the central nervous system feeding pathway (*15*). Recently, it has been discovered that adipocytes secrete a large number of proteases. Some of these have been suggested to be relatively adipocyte specific. Of these, the serine protease named adipsin has been suggested as a putative regulatory signal to the central nervous system. Adipsin was originally derived from cDNA probes developed in the laboratory of Spiegelman and associates (*16*). Adipsin is lacking in several genetically obese animal models such as the *ob/ob* and the *db/db* mouse (*17*). While its biological function is still unclear, this representative of new adipocyte messages may prove a useful tool for further understanding the relationship between energy stores at the adipocyte level and feeding behavior.

SUMMARY

Studies of adipose tissue cellularity in experimental animals have revealed that adipocyte number may be increased at any age. This can occur in response to a high sucrose diet. There is also increasing evidence that there are regional differences in adipose tissue metabolsm that have significant impact on some of the health risks associated with obesity. In comparison to lower body obesity ("pear" shape), upper body obesity ("apple" shape) is associated with increased risk for diabetes, heart disease, and hypertension. Finally, although food intake may be influenced by adipose tissue-derived signals, to-date these have not been elucidated. An attractive candidate for this role is adipsin—which is lacking in several geneticall obese animal models.

REFERENCES

1. Knittle, J.L. and Hirsch, J. (1968). Effect of early nutrition on the development of rat epididymal fat pads: Cellularity and metabolism. *J. Clin. Invest.* **47**, 2091–2120.
2. Johnson, P.R., Stern, J.S., Greenwood, M.R.C., Zucker, L.M., and Hirsch, J. (1973). Effect of early nutrition on adipose cellularity and pancreatic insulin release in the Zucker rat. *J. Nutr.* **103**, 738–743.
3. Faust, I.M., Johnson, P.R., Stern, J.S., and Hirsch, J. (1978). Diet-induced adipocyte number increase in adult rats: A new model of obesity. *Am. J. Physiol.* **235**, R279–R286.
4. Ellis, J.R., McDonald, R.B., and Stern, J.S. (1987). Effect of diet on adipocyte proliferation in older rats. *Fed. Proc.* **46**, 881.
5. Stern, J.S., Titchenal, C.A., and Johnson, P.R. (1987). Obesity: does exercise make a difference. *In* "Recent Advances in Obesity Research," Berry, E.M., Blondheim, S.H., Eliahou, H.E., and Shafrir, E., eds., pp. 337–349. John Libby, London.
6. Walberg, J.L., Mole, P.A., and Stern, J.S. (1982). Effect of swim training on development of obesity in the genetically obese rat. *Am. J. Physiol.* **242**, R204–R211.
7. Applegate, E.A. and Stern, J.S. (1987). Exercise termination effects on food intake, plasma insulin, and adipose lipoprotein lipase activity in the Osborne-Mendel rat. *Metabolism* **36**, 709–714.
8. Ellis, J.R. and Stern, J.S. The effect of cessation of exercise on fat cell proliferation, in preparation.
9. Rebuffe-Scrive, M., Lonnroth, P., Marin, P., Wesslau, C., Bjorntorp, P., and Smith, U. (1987). Regional adipose tissue metabolism in men and post-menopausal women. *Int. J. Obesity* **11**, 347–355.
10. Rebuffe-Scrive, M., Eldh, J., Hafstron, L., and Bjorntorp, P. (1986). Metabolism of mammary, abdominal, and femoral adipocytes in women before and after menopause. *Metabolism* **35**, 792–797.
11. Rebuffe-Scrive, M., Enk, L., Crona, N., Lonnroth, P., Abrahamsson, L., Smith, U., and Bjorntorp, P. (1985). Fat cell metabolism in different regions in women. *J. Clin. Invest.* **75**, 1973–1976.
12. Steingrimsdottir, L.J., Brasel, J., and Greenwood, M.R.C. (1980). Hormonal

modulation on adipose tissue lipoprotein lipase may alter food intake in rats. *Am. J. Physiol.* **239**, E167–180.

13. Wade, G.N. and Gray, J. (1976). Sex hormones, regulatory behaviors, and body weight. *In* "Advances in the Study of Behavior," Rosenblatt, J.S., Hinde, R.A., Shaw, E., and Beer, C.G., eds., Vol. 6, pp. 201–279. Academic Press, New York.
14. Kissebah, A.H., Vydelingum, N., Murray, R., Evans, D.J., Hartz, A.J., Kalkhoff, R.K., and Adams, P.W. (1982). Relation of body fat distribution to metabolic complications of obesity. *J. Clin. Endocrinol. Metab.* **54**, 254–260.
15. Faust, I.M. (1984). The role of the fat cell in energy balance physiology. *In* "Eating and Its Disorders," Stunkard, A.J. and Stellar, E., eds., pp. 97–107. Raven Press, New York.
16. Spiegelman, B.M., Frank, M., and Green, H. (1983). Molecular cloning of mRNA from 3T3 adipocytes. *J. Biol. Chem.* **258**, 10083–10089.
17. Flier, J.S., Cool, K.S., Usher, P., and Spiegelman, B.M. (1987). Severely impaired adipsin expression in genetic and acquired obesity. *Science* **237**, 405–408.

Diet and Obesity, Bray, G.A. *et al.*, eds., pp. 181–190.
Japan Sci. Soc. Press, Tokyo/S. Karger, Basel (1988)

Exercise Training and Energy Expenditure

JACQUES LeBLANC

Department of Physiology, School of Medicine, Laval University, Quebec P.Q., G1K 7P4, Canada

Physical activity is an important factor in the control of body weight. Considering the effect of exercise *per se* the energy expenditure associated with the cost of various exercises may have large influence on energy balance. In addition, the habit of exercise, at levels corresponding to $\simeq$60% and above, of maximum oxygen consumption, ($\dot{V}O_{2\,max}$) leads to adaptive responses which allow a person to gradually increase the amount of work, and the corresponding energy expenditure, for an activity equivalent to the same percentage of $\dot{V}O_{2\,max}$. In other words, for the same effort, the oxygen consumption may be significantly augmented and as a result the habit of exercising gradually increase the energy expenditure. Another advantage associated with physical activity is the increase in energy expenditure for many hours following the cessation of activity. This has been termed excess post-exercise oxygen consumption (EPOC) (*1*). A recent study investigated the effect of exercise at 70% of $\dot{V}O_{2\,max}$ for 20, 40 or 80 min on EPOC and on meal induced thermogenesis (*2*). After exercising 80 min, EPOC was increased by 15% over a period of 12 hr (Fig. 1). The authors

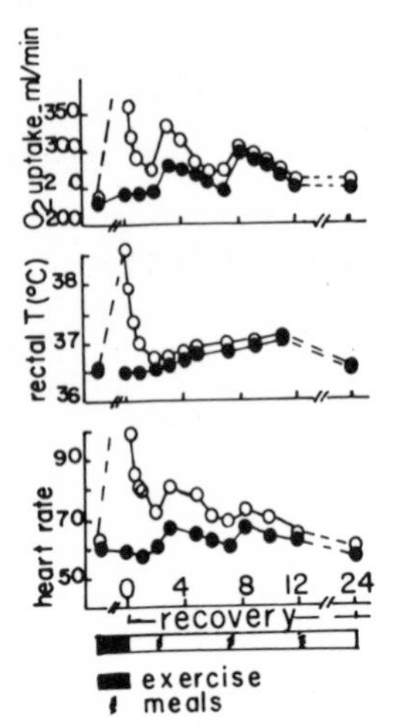

Fig. 1. Effects of 80 min exercise on EPOC, on rectal temperature and heart rate during the 24 hr period following exercise (*2*).

proposed that EPOC is due to increased rates of "futile" substrate cycling possibly caused by an increased activity of the sympathetic nervous system and by the cost of glycogen synthesis (*1, 3, 4*). It also seems likely that such physiological functions as heart rate, ventilation and especially body temperature (*5*) which remain elevated for some time after exercise, could also be involved in the maintenance of EPOC. In summary, EPOC increases energy expenditures more than could be expected from the cost of exercise *per se*. It should be mentioned that EPOC was not observed with aerobic work corresponding to 30–50% of $\dot{V}O_{2\,max}$ (*6*). The fact that EPOC is observed only with anaerobic exercise (*7*) suggests the possible participation of the sympathetic nervous system since this system is activated at about the same level of activity (*8*).

I. EXERCISE AND DIETING

Another thermogenic action of exercise has been recently described in association with dieting for the treatment of obesity. Resting metabolic rate (RMR) and body weight changes were

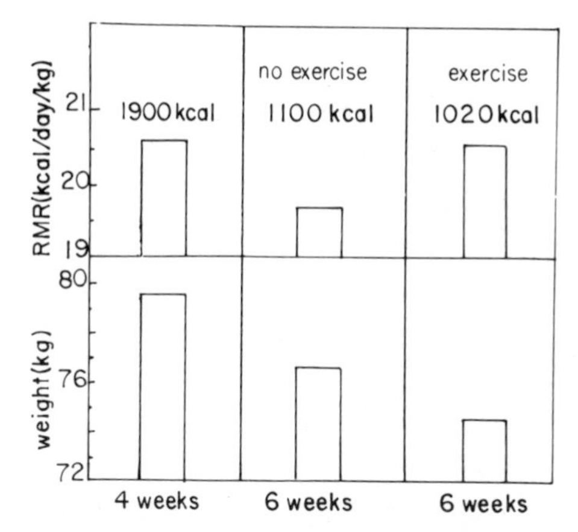

Fig. 2. Body weight and RMR in subjects fed either 1,900 kcal, 1,100 kcal or 1,020 kcal associated with an exercise program during a period of 6 weeks (*9*).

measured over an 18 week period in ten overweight women (*9*). It was confirmed that body weight reduction caused by dieting declines gradually as the period of caloric restriction is extended (*10*). This adaptive phenomenon would seem to be related to a significant reduction of RMR. It was also found that exercise when associated with caloric restriction caused an elevation of RMR to predieting levels (*9*) (Fig. 2). Thus, in addition to an increase in energy expenditure caused by physical activity, exercise favors weight loss by increasing RMR. The effect of exercise is added to that of dieting and potentiates its action on weight loss. This study also raised the question of the effect of exercise on body weight control and adiposity. Results from a bank of subjects engaged in various sports in the Department of Physical Education at Laval University confirm observations reported by others (*11*). A very significant negative correlation is found between the percentage of fat and the $\dot{V}O_{2\,max}$ (Fig. 3). When the subjects are regrouped by sex and by levels of $\dot{V}O_{2\,max}$, the results show that for the same level of training, the adiposity of women is higher than that of men. The reduced adiposity of highly trained subjects indicates that they had been in a negative energy balance and that the caloric intake had

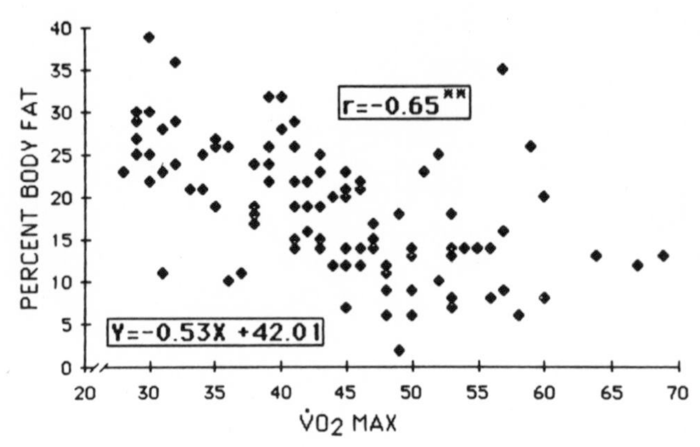

Fig. 3. Influence of level of training ($\dot{V}O_{2\,max}$) on percentage of body fat (*11*).

been somewhat reduced. In order to further elucidate this question, a series of experiments was done on rats in which complete energy balance measurements were made (*12*). When male rats are made to exercise daily for 1.5 hr for a period of 30 days, the total energy intake is reduced, causing a diminution of total energy gain and of body weight gain which are explained by a reduction of about 50% of both body protein and body fat gain compared to control sedentary rats. The analysis of complete energy balance shows that the reduced energy intake of the trained rats is totally accounted for by the reduced energy gain and the added cost of exercise; there is no difference in energy expenditure which could suggest a regulatory adaptive metabolic effect of exercise training (Table I). Yet EPOC has been described in rats as well as in humans (*25*). Perhaps the absence of noticeable action of EPOC in this chronic study is explained by some opposite effect of exercise on energy expenditure. One can suggest as a possibility the greater inactivity as a result of strenuous exercise in the trained rats when compared to sedentary rats. When sedentary and trained rats are fed palatable high fat diet the energy intake is increased by 30% and 20%, respectively. This excess energy is totally explained by body fat gain in both groups. The protein deposition is not changed by overfeeding (Fig. 4). This means that the 40% reduction of protein gain found in exercise-

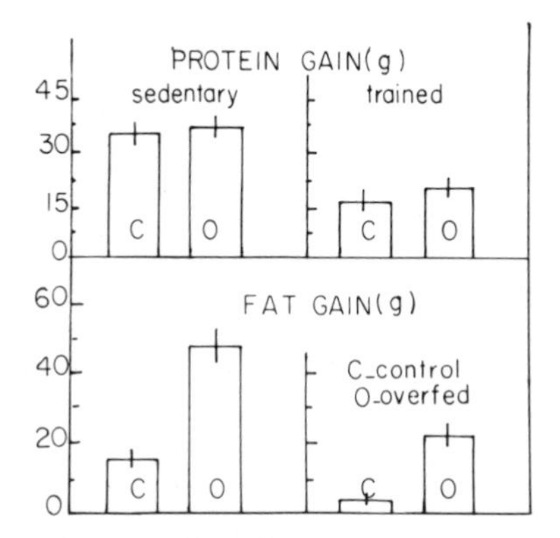

Fig. 4. Effect of exercise training on fat and protein gain of rats fed standard laboratory chow or cafeteria diet (*12*).

trained rats fed standard laboratory chow is also found when these animals are overfed (*13*). Thus the reduction of protein synthesis observed in exercise-trained male rats is not due to caloric deprivation but instead to some factor directly related to the exercise. It is interesting to note that this effect of training on growth is not observed in female rats (*14*). Considering the fact that plasma levels of testosterone are reduced by exercise training (*15*), it is tempting to suggest that the diminution of androgens, a hormone which stimulates protein synthesis, might explain the reduction of protein gain in exercise-trained male rats. This question remains to be elucidated since the plasma level of other hormones, such as triiodothyronine which are involved in protein synthesis has also been shown to be diminished during exercise-training in rats (*16*). The whole of these results also suggests an effect of exercise on appetite, especially in males. The mechanism of this action, however, is not known.

II. EXERCISE AND METABOLIC RATE

Another aspect of exercise with relation to energy expenditure concerns the effect of exercise-training on RMR and on meal-induced thermogenesis. Many studies have reported a significant

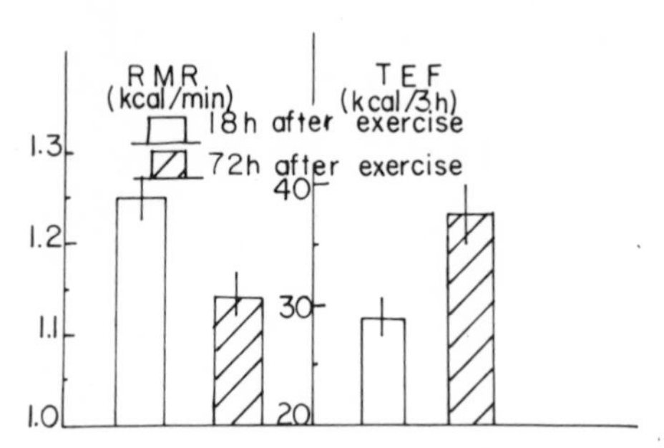

Fig. 5. RMR and TEF either 18 or 72 hr after the last bout of exercise in highly trained subjects (*18*).

elevation of RMR in trained compared to untrained subjects. This action was observed in highly trained athletes with $VO_{2\ max}$ between 65 and 75 ml/kg/min (*17–19*). Some investigators failed to confirm this finding (*20, 21*). In these latter studies, the $VO_{2\ max}$ of the subjects indicate low to moderate levels of training. It is also interesting to note that RMR of trained subjects measured 3 days after the last bout of exercise is not different from that of untrained subjects (*18*) (Fig. 5). These studies show that the increase in RMR, which is caused by high levels of exercise is rapidly reversed during a detraining period. The reasons for these actions are not known. The thermic effect of feeding (TEF) has also been shown to be influenced by the level of training. Reports have indicated that TEF is reduced by approximately 30 to 50% in trained compared to untrained subjects (*17, 19, 22, 23*). In all these studies, TEF was measured about 16 hr after the last bout of exercise. When the rest period is increased to 36 hr or more, the results show the same or even increased thermogenesis in response to a meal in trained compared to non-trained subjects (*20, 21*). This is well illustrated by Tremblay *et al.* (*18*) who have shown a reduced TEF in trained subjects when measurements were made 3 days after the last bout of exercise as opposed to 16 hr (Fig. 5). Thus RMR is increased and the TEF is decreased in the immediate hours that follow exercise, but these same variables resume normal responses when the subjects have been inactive for 3 days or more. The reduced TEF in trained

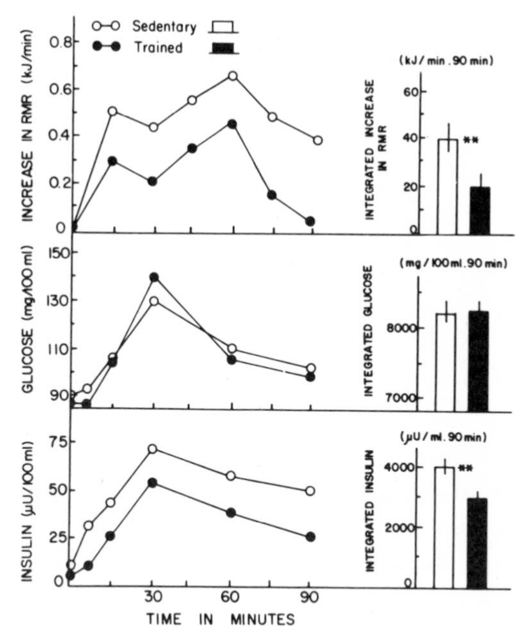

Fig. 6. Effect of a standard meal on RMR, plasma glucose, and insulin of sedentary and highly trained subjects (*22*).

subjects is possibly related to some hormonal influence since both the plasma insulin and norepinephrine responses to a meal are significantly reduced in these subjects compared to untrained subjects (*22, 24*) (Fig. 6). We have suggested that the reduced insulin requirements of trained subjects in response to glucose intake could be explained by a larger transformation into glycogen, a process also requiring less energy than storage in the form of fat (*24*). This was indirectly confirmed by Tremblay *et al.* who reported a concomitant increase in glucose storage and a reduced thermic effect in trained subjects fed 75g of glucose (*18*) (Fig. 7).

In conclusion, we can say that in addition to directly increasing energy expenditure, exercise would seem to potentiate the weight reducing action of dieting. Also, the habit of exercise for many people is a source of pleasure and satisfaction which is usually not

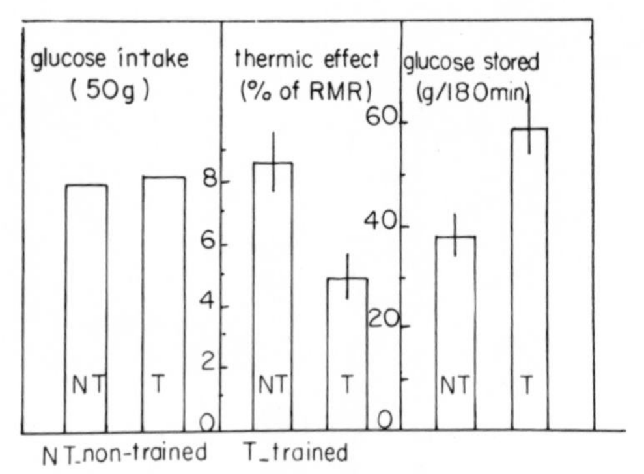

Fig. 7. Glucose storage and thermic effect of feeding 50 g glucose to trained and non-trained human subjects (*18*).

encountered when a program of dieting is followed. For these reasons, the combination of exercise and dieting would seem to be the best method for achieving successful body weight reduction and control.

SUMMARY

In a large group of young population, the percentage of body fat is found to be inversely proportional to the intensity of physical activity in which they are engaged. This finding indicates that the increased energy intake for a given level of physical activity is not proportional to the level of energy expenditure. There are indications as well that excess energy is consumed in the hours that follow exercise, especially if it has been intense. It is concluded that the association of motivated exercise and dieting is the best means of exerting fruitful control of body weight.

REFERENCES

1. Gaesser, G.A. and Brooks, G.A. (1984). Metabolic bases of excess post-exercise oxygen consumption: a review. *Med. Sci. Sports Med.* **16**, 29-44.
2. Bahr, R., Ingnes, I., Vaage, O., Sejersted, O.M., and Newsholme, E.A. (1987).

Effect of duration of exercise on excess post-exercise O_2 consumption. *J. Appl. Physiol.* **62**, 485–490.

3. Hermansen, L., Grandmontagne, M., Maehlum, S., and Ingnes, L. (1984). Postexercise elevation of resting oxygen uptake: possible mechanisms and physiological significance. *In* "Physiological Chemistry of Training and Detraining," pp. 119–129. Karger, Basel.
4. Allborg, G. and Felig, P. (1982). Lactate and glucose exchange across the forearm, legs and splanchnic bed during and after prolonged leg exercise. *J. Clin. Invest.* **69**, 45–54.
5. Brooks, G.A., Hittelman, K.J., Faulkner, J.A., and Bayer, R.E. (1971). Temperature, skeletal muscle mitochondrial functions, and oxygen debt. *Am. J. Physiol.* **220**, 1053–1059.
6. Pacy, P.J., Barton, N., Webster, J., and Garrow, J.S. (1985). The energy cost of aerobic exercise in fed and fasted normal subjects. *Am. J. Clin. Nutr.* **42**, 764–768.
7. Brehm, B. and Gutin, B. (1986). Recovery energy expenditure for steady state exercise in runners and non exercisers. *Med. Sci. Sports Exercise* **18**, 205–210.
8. Galbo, H., Holst, J.J., and Christensen, N.J. (1976). Glucagon plasma catecholamine responses to graded and prolonged exercise in man. *J. Appl. Physiol.* **38**, 70–76.
9. Donahoe, G.P., Lin, D.H., Kirschenbaum, D.S., and Keesey, R.E. (1984). Metabolic consequences of dieting and exercise in the treatment of obesity. *J. Consult. Clin. Psychol.* **52**, 827–836.
10. Apfelbaum, M. (1978). Adaptation to changes in caloric intake. *Prog. Food Nutr. Sci.* **2**, 543–559.
11. LeBlanc, J., Tremblay, A., and Bouchard, C. Unpublished data.
12. Richard, D., Arnold, J., and LeBlanc, J. (1986). Energy balance in exercise-trained rats acclimated at two environmental temperatures. *J. Appl. Physiol.* **60**, 1054–1059.
13. Arnold, J. and Richard, D. (1987). Unaltered regulatory thermogenic response to dietary signals in exercise-trained rats. *Am. J. Physiol.* **252**, R617–R623.
14. LeBlanc, J., Dussault, J., Lupien, D., and Richard, D. (1982). Effect of diet and exercise on norepinephrine-induced thermogenesis in male and female rats. *J. Appl. Physiol.* **52**, 556–561.
15. Wheeler, G.D., Wall, S.R., Belcastro, A.N., and Cumming, D.C. (1984). Reduced serum testosterone levels in male distance runners. *JAMA* **252**, 514–516.
16. LeBlanc, J., Labrie, A., Lupien, D., and Richard, D. (1982). Catecholamines and triiodothyronine variations and the calorigenic response to norepinephrine in cold-adapted and exercise-trained rats. *Can. J. Physiol. Pharmacol.* **60**, 783–787.
17. LeBlanc, J., Jobin, M., Côté, J., Samson, P., and Labrie, A. (1985). Enhanced metabolic response to caffeine in exercise-trained subjects. *J. Appl. Physiol.* **59**, 832–837.
18. Tremblay, A., Fontaine, E., and Nadeau, A. (1985). Contribution of post exercise increment in glucose storage to variations in glucose-induced thermogenesis in

endurance athletes. *Can J. Physiol. Pharmacol.* **63**, 1165-1169.

19. Tremblay, A., Fontaine, E., Pochlman, E.T., Mitchell, D., Perron, L., and Bouchard, C. (1986). The effect of exercise-training on resting metabolic rate in lean and moderately obese individuals. *Int. J. Obesity* **10**, 511-517.
20. Hill, J.O., Heymsfield, S.B., McMannus, C., and DiGirolamo, M. (1984). Meal size and thermic response to food in male subjects as a function of maximum aerobic capacity. *Metabolism* **33**, 742-749.
21. Davis, J.R., Tagliaferro, A.R., Kertzer, R., Gerardo, T., Nichols, J., and Wheeler, J. (1983). Variations in dietary-induced thermogenesis and body fatness with aerobic capacity. *Eur. J. Appl. Physiol.* **19**, 1051-1055.
22. LeBlanc, J., Diamond, P., Côté, J., and A. Labrie (1974). Hormonal factor in reduced postprandial heat production of exercise-trained subjects. *J. Appl. Physiol.* **56**, 772-776.
23. LeBlanc, J., Mercier, P., and Samson, P. (1984). Diet-induced thermogenesis with relation to training state in female subjects. *Can. J. Physiol. Pharmacol.* **62**, 334-337.
24. LeBlanc, J., Nadeau, A., Richard, D., and Tremblay, A. (1981). Studies on the sparing effect of exercise on insulin requirements in human subjects. *Metabolism* **30**, 1119-1125.
25. Gleeson, M., Brown, J.F., Waring, J.J., and Stock, M.J. (1981). The effects of physical exercise on metabolic rate and dietary-induced thermogenesis. *Br. J. Nutr.* **47**, 173-182.

Diet and Obesity, Bray, G.A. et al., eds., pp. 191-204.
Japan Sci. Soc. Press, Tokyo/S. Karger, Basel (1988)

Roles of Dietary Fat, Carbohydrate Balance and Exercise in the Regulation of Body Weight

JEAN-PIERRE FLATT

Department of Biochemistry, University of Massachusetts Medical School, Worcester, MA 01655, U.S.A.

Body weights are usually stable over prolonged periods. This weight maintenance situation, in which energy expenditure varies about the same mean as energy intake, can only be sustained if protein, carbohydrate and fat balances are each achieved. Appreciable deviations from exact balances undoubtedly occur from day to day, but it appears that depletion or accumulation of body constituents must somehow elicit corrective responses. These may manifest themselves by influencing food intake, and by altering the rate of energy expenditure or the composition of the substrate mix used for energy generation. Thanks to these responses, the oxidative disposal of amino acids, glucose and fatty acids can be made to occur at rates corresponding, in the average, to the proportions of protein, carbohydrate and fat present in the diet.

The need to properly adjust the composition of the fuel mix used for energy generation presents constraints beyond the mere need to achieve energy balance. The size of the body's protein pools, the state of repletion of its glycogen reserves, and the volume of the adipose tissue mass, all influence the concentrations of circulating substrates and hormones and, thereby, the rates of substrate utilization. Changes in body composition thus contribute to the adjustment of the fuel mix oxidized to the nutrient distribution in the diet, and the particular body composition must be reached for which the fuel mixture oxidized has the same average composition as the diet consumed (*1*). The composition of the diet is thus a factor, along with genetic traits, dietary habits and life style in determining for which body composition weight maintenance will be achieved (*2, 3*).

I. SUBSTRATE BALANCES

Adjustment of amino acid oxidation to protein intake is effectively achieved since nitrogen balance (or a stable rate of protein accretion during growth) is maintained on high or low (but adequate) protein intakes, irrespective of the ratio of carbohydrate-to-fat in the diet. In view of this, and because carbohydrate and fat provide the bulk of energy substrates used for ATP generation, weight maintenance is determined primarily by events pertaining to the metabolism of carbohydrates and fats. Carbohydrate and fat can both provide substrates for ATP generation. The regulation of their metabolism differs substantially, however. In mice maintained *ad libitum* on diets of fixed composition, for instance, carbohydrate oxidation is positively correlated with daily food and carbohydrate intake, whereas fat oxidation is negatively correlated with food and fat intake (*cf.* Flatt, this book). Thus carbohydrate intake promotes its oxidation, whereas fat intake does not. This reflects the fact that the body's fat stores contain about 100 times more energy than can be stored as glycogen, and that biological evolution was therefore compelled to lead to the development of mechanisms (including hormonal responses) that give priority to the maintenance of the carbohydrate balance over that of the fat balance. This priority is further illustrated by the adjustment in daily food intake observed among *ad libitum* fed mice (Fig. 1). The negative correlation between changes in food intake from one day to the other and the previous day's carbohydrate and fat balances is much steeper in the

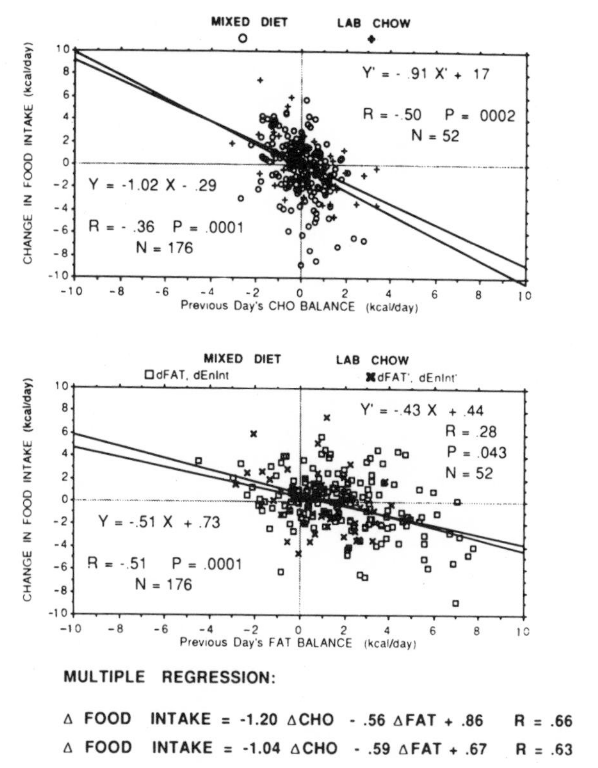

Fig. 1. Changes in food intake in relation to the previous day's carbohydrate and fat balances in 12 *ad libitum* fed mice monitored continuously over periods of 14 or 24 days. Daily carbohydrate and fat balances were established from the weight of food consumed per day, the nutrient of the diets, and the amounts of carbohydrate and fat oxidized over 24 hr, as determined by indirect calorimetry. Changes in food intake correspond to differences in the energy intake of individual mice observed over 2 consecutive 24-hr periods. For further experimental details see Flatt, this book.

case of carbohydrate. These correlations are remarkably similar among mice maintained on lab chow or on a mixed diet. Assuming that these relationships are indicative of a negative feedback regulation in the control of food intake, one finds that the effect of deviations from the fat balance on food intake, while tending to reduce the size of the imbalance, is not sufficient to correct for errors

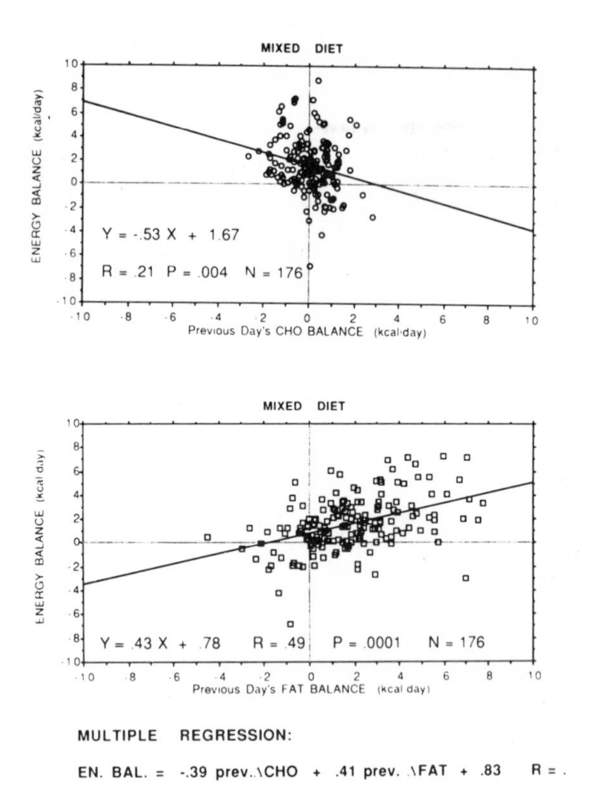

Fig. 2. Daily energy balances in relation to the previous day's carbohydrate and fat balances in *ad libitum* fed mice. For experimental conditions see legend to Fig. 1.

in the overall energy balance (Fig. 2). The data indicate that a fat imbalance tends to be part of a trend which manifests itself over several consecutive days. In sharp contrast, the apparent response to errors in the carbohydrate balance does tend to cause a reversal of the energy imbalance, in a manner capable of promoting the maintenance of energy balance (Fig. 2).

II. STEADY STATE OF WEIGHT MAINTENANCE

The very large difference in storage capacities for carbohydrate and for fat has implications as well for the body's ability to achieve the steady state of weight maintenance. This can be appreciated with the help of a model comprising two reservoirs of very different capacities (Fig. 3). The small reservoir is meant to represent the body's limited capacity for storing glycogen, whereas the large reservoir corresponds to the body's ability to store large amounts of fat. (The units used in Fig. 3 were chosen to be roughly equivalent to the body's glycogen and fat reserves, in terms of kcal.) The contributions made by the small and by the large reservoir to the flux of turbine A (see upper right panel) are assumed to occur in proportion to the hydrostatic pressures prevailing in the two reservoirs. Replenishment occurs from time to time; the fraction of the total fuel added which falls into the large reservoir corresponds, in this analogy, to the fat content of the diet. Given the large cross-sectional area of the large reservoir, the amount of fuel added during one "outflow-replenishment cycle" will cause only an insignificant change in its level. Changes in its content, therefore, do not provide a favorable site of origin for signals that could be used to trigger fuel replenishment at appropriate intervals. On the other hand, changes in the fuel level in the small reservoir are very marked, much more likely to be detectable, and more suitable to trigger replenishment at appropriate intervals. It is thus assumed in the model that fuel addition is elicited whenever the content of the small reservoir has dropped to a particular minimal level. The cumulative effects of repeated imbalances between additions and outflow can, in time, lead to substantial changes in the content of the large reservoir. Ultimately, the situation will be encountered in which the hydrostatic pressure in the large reservoir will be just right to cause the outflow from it during one cycle to be equal to the amount of fuel added to it. Subsequently, replenishment triggered at a frequency which serves to maintain the content of the small reservoir in its operating range will cause no further accumulation or depletion in the large reservoir. A steady state is then reached which will tend to maintain itself. It is noteworthy that the level in the large reservoir establishes itself at a particular height, without there being a sensor to measure its content nor any mechanism that

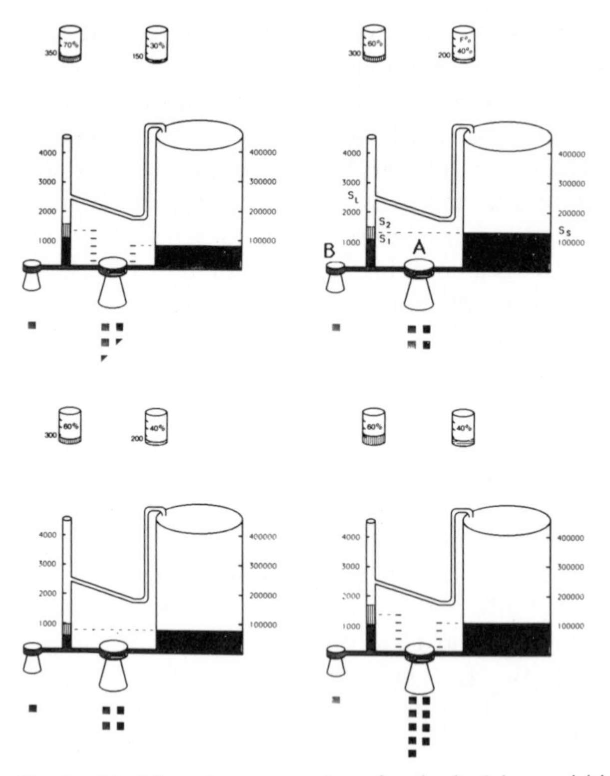

Fig. 3. Model used as an analogy for the body's acquisition, storage and oxidation of carbohydrate (small reservoir) and of fat (large reservoir). (Units were chosen to correspond to the body's glycogen and fat reserves, expressed in kcal). Turbine A (see upper right panel) is fed by the two reservoirs, which contribute to its flux in amounts proportional to the hydrostatic pressures prevailing in the two reservoirs at a given time. The power output from turbine A is variable (representative of physical Activity changes). Turbine B is fed only from the small reservoir and its outflow is constant (analogy with the Brain's requirement for glucose). When the water level in the small reservoir declines to level S_1 a given mass of water M (analogy for a Meal) is added to the system, of which a fraction F (corresponding to the Fat content of the diet) falls into the large reservoir, the remainder being added to the small reservoir. When water accumulates to a sufficient height in the small reservoir (S_L) it can be transferred into the large reservoir, to mimic lipogenesis from carbohydrate. (Under usual conditions, glycogen reserves remain below the level (*i.e.*, about 8 g/kg body weight) needed to induce a rate of lipogenesis exceeding the

could drive the system to some predetermined set-point value. (For a more detailed analysis of the model see ref. *3*).

III. EFFECT OF DIETARY FAT CONTENT

In the two upper and the lower left panel of Fig. 3, 20% of total flux is assumed to occur through turbine B (*i.e.*, the same proportion as the brain's glucose expenditure in the resting state). Changes in the proportion of fuel added to the two reservoirs will cause shifts in their steady state levels. For example, if 40% of the added fuel falls into the large reservoir (upper right panel), the level achieved therein will become stable when the two reservoirs contribute equally to the flux through turbine A, considering that one third of the fuel added to the small reservoir (*i.e.*, 20% of the total fuel added) escapes through turbine B. The level in the large reservoir thus establishes itself at a height exerting a hydrostatic pressure equal to the average hydrostatic pressure prevailing in the small reservoir. If only 30% of the fuel added falls into the large reservoir (upper left panel), its steady state level will be lower, corresponding to 3/5 of the average level in the small reservoir. The two upper panels of Fig. 3 thus illustrate that increments in the fraction of fuel falling into the large reservoir cause an increase in its steady state level, as long as the level which triggers replenishment in the small reservoir remains unchanged. However, such an increase can be prevented by changing the height for which replenishment is triggered, as shown in the lower left panel. With regard to the regulation of body weight, these examples thus illustrate that the range within which glycogen levels are maintained must be lowered, if an expansion of the adipose tissue mass is to be avoided when the fat content of the diet increases.

The constant availability of palatable foods may tend to prevent a reduction of sufficient magnitude in the range within which glycogen reserves are spontaneously maintained, to permit a rate of

---

concomittant rate of fat oxidation (*4*). L_S) indicates the large reservoir when steady state conditions have become established; four such steady state situations are illustrated (see text).

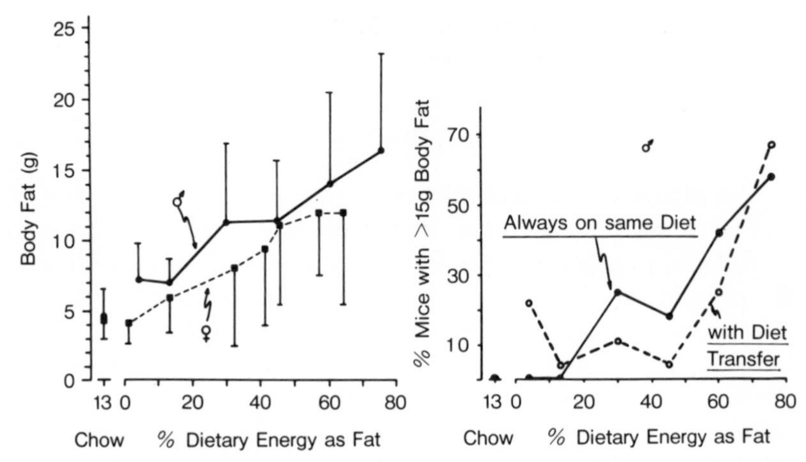

Fig. 4. Effect of the diet's fat content on the body fat content and on the incidence of obesity among *ad libitum* fed mice. The points shown at left are means ± SEM; their position along the abscissa indicates the fat content of the diet provided at the time of sacrifice (protein contents = 18% of total energy). 133 female (■) and 71 male CDl mice (●) were maintained constantly on the same diet; another 100 male mice (0) were transferred for the last 2-3 months to high, or low fat diets after being maintained previously on low, or high fat diets, respectively. Reproduced with permission from ref. *2*.

fat oxidation commensurate with the diet's fat content without expansion of the adipose tissue mass. Indeed, among *ad libitum* fed mice maintained on diets in which the fat-to-carbohydrate ratio is raised, one observes a gradual increase in the average body fat content (Fig. 4) (*2*).

IV. POST-PRANDIAL *VERSUS* POST-ABSORPTIVE FUEL OXIDATION

In the body, as in the model, the fuel mix oxidized after a meal is influenced by the amounts of carbohydrate consumed, but not by the amount of fat provided by the meal. This is demonstrated by the observation that glucose, insulin, and free fatty acid (FFA) concentrations, as well as the respiratory quotient (RQ), exhibit the same postprandial time-course after breakfasts supplying identical

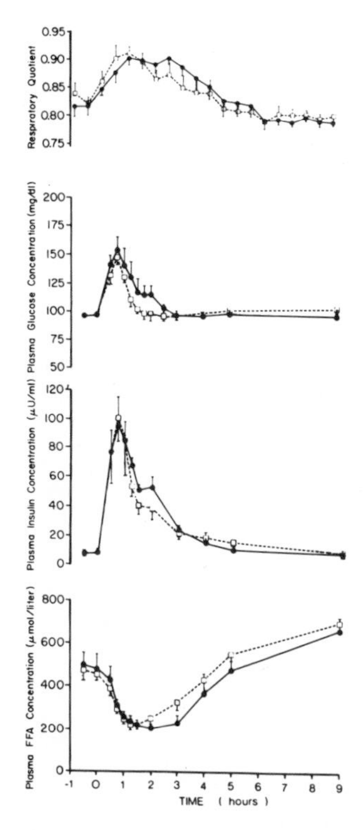

Fig. 5. Changes in the non-protein-RQ and in blood glucose, plasma insulin, and FFA concentrations in response to a low fat breakfast (●) containing 75 g of light bread, 72 g of jam, and 60 g of dry meat (73 g of carbohydrate, 6 g of fat, and 30 g of protein) and after the same breakfast supplemented with 50 g margarine (□) that provided an additional 41 g of fat. Means±SEM. Reprinted with permission from ref. *5*.

amounts of carbohydrate and protein, but different amounts of fat (Fig. 5) (*5*). The nutrient composition of the fat-supplemented test meal was chosen to be identical to the substrate mix used for energy production in the post-absorptive state. Thus, the prompt increase in the subjects' RQ shows by itself that metabolic regulation in man also gives a higher priority to the maintenance of carbohydrate balance over that of fat balance. Evidently, the contribution made by lipids to the fuel mix used for energy generation is determined by

TABLE I
Effects of Exercise on Post-absorptive Metabolic Rate and RQ (*9*)

		RQ	BMR	CHOoxid	FAToxid
	Day 1:	0.85 ± 0.01	1.37 ± 0.05	0.60	0.56
				(44%)	(41%)
ΔGlycogen = −49 g		($p < .001$)	($p < .05$)		
ΔFat = −36 g					
ΔProtein = +41 g					
	Day 2:	0.81 ± 0.01	1.44 ± 0.06	0.45	0.78
				(31%)	(54%)

Bielinski *et al.* (*9*) studied a group of athletic young men in a respiratory chamber. Measurements of their metabolism in the post-absorptive state were made on two consecutive mornings, separated by a day that included 3 hr of walking on a treadmill at 50% of the subjects' $\dot{V}O_{2\,max}$. The decrease in their glycogen levels appears to provide an explanation for the observed decrease in their RQ. Such an effect may exert a greater effect on steady-state conditions of weight maintenance that the small increment in their basal metabolic rate.

other factors than the amount of fat just ingested. These factors include the availability of FFA, which is regulated by insulin. Short-term changes in insulin secretion are controlled by carbohydrate intake and explain why fat oxidation decreases after a meal, regardless of its fat content (see RQ changes in Fig. 5). FFA levels are also influenced, albeit to a much lesser extent, by the size of an individual's adipose tissue mass (*6*), which reflects the cumulative effect of long sustained fat imbalances. The development of insulin resistance when the adipose tissue mass becomes excessive further contributes to enhance the oxidation of fat relative to carbohydrate (*7*). The model thus provides a rationale to explain why an expansion of the adipose tissue can facilitate the approach to a steady state of weight maintenance in individuals who appear to be unable to maintain energy balance while lean.

V. EFFECTS OF EXERCISE

The two right-hand panels in Fig. 3 illustrate that a change in the flux through turbine A, while outflow through turbine B is constant, also alters the conditions for which the steady state

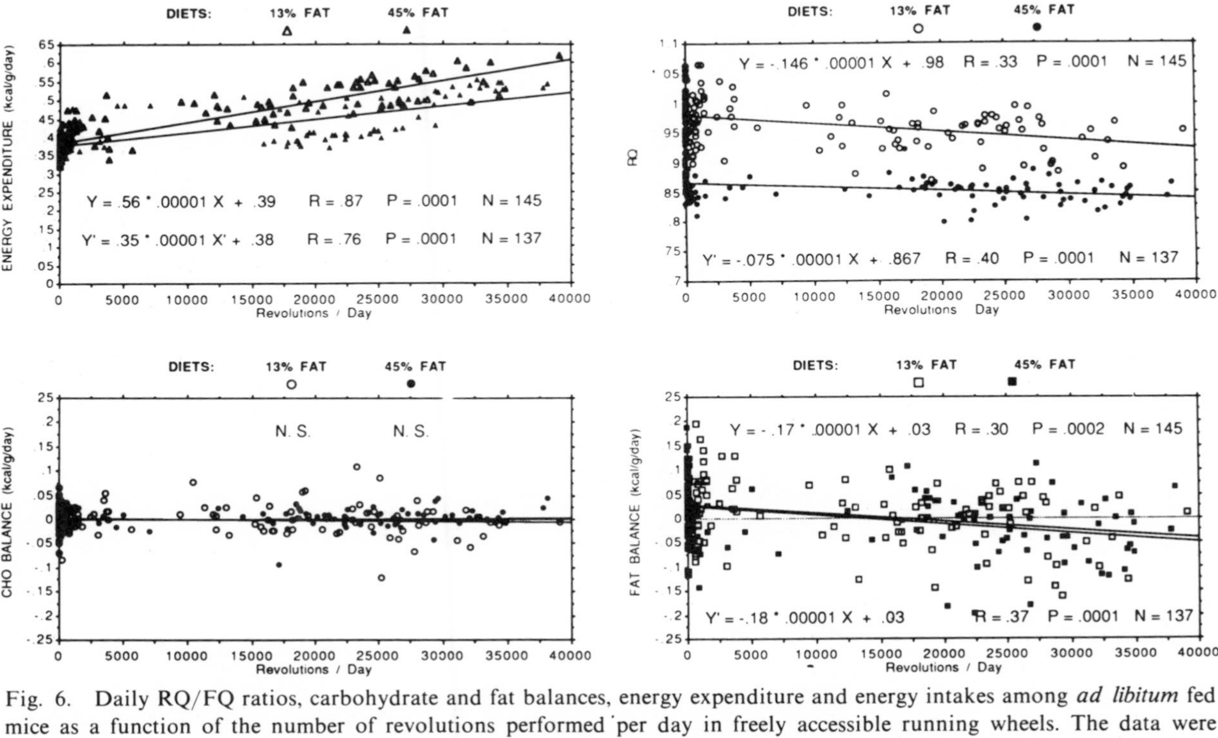

Fig. 6. Daily RQ/FQ ratios, carbohydrate and fat balances, energy expenditure and energy intakes among *ad libitum* fed mice as a function of the number of revolutions performed per day in freely accessible running wheels. The data were obtained in 10 female CDl mice monitored continuously over a 29 day period. Their diets contained 18% of energy as protein, 13% or 45% as fat, and 69% or 37% carbohydrate. Experimental conditions were similar to those described in the legend to Fig. 1.

becomes established. With a doubling of total flux (lower right panel), the drain on the small reservoir caused by turbine B decreases from 20% to 10% of total flux, thereby increasing the outflow through turbine A, which is alimented by both reservoirs. A lesser hydrostatic pressure in the large reservoir is then sufficient to reach steady-state conditions. (In the absence of turbine B, the model's behavior would not be affected by changes in total flux rate, *cf.* ref. *3.*)

In the resting state, a substantial fraction of total energy expenditure occurs in tissues which use glucose exclusively. Increases in total energy expenditure caused by exercise lead to increased fuel oxidation in muscle, which burns FFA as well as glucose. The gradual decline in the RQ during prolonged exercise shows that depletion of the body's glycogen reserves during (*8*) (as well as after prolonged exertion (Table I) (*9*)) further contributes to promote the use of fat as a metabolic fuel. In *ad libitum* fed mice which have free access to a running wheel, increased exertion is associated with a reduction in the RQ and negative fat balances (Fig. 6). The increment in food intake elicited by increased exercise, though sufficient to maintain carbohydrate balance, will not fully compensate for the increase in energy expenditure (Fig. 6). When substantial amounts of physical activity are part of the daily routine, the steady state of weight maintenance can therefore be attained without (or with a lesser) expansion of the adipose tissue mass, even when mixed diets with substantial fat contents are consumed.

SUMMARY

Weight maintenance requires that the fuel mix oxidized has the same carbohydrate-to-fat ratio as the diet. This can be stated by saying that the average RQ must be equal to the "food quotient" or "FQ" of the diet (*1*) (the "FQ" being defined as the ratio of CO_2 produced to O_2 consumption during the oxidation of a representative sample of the diet). This is illustrated by the data in Fig. 7, which show that energy balance is achieved when the RQ/FQ ratio is equal to one, regardless of the composition of the diet. Multiple

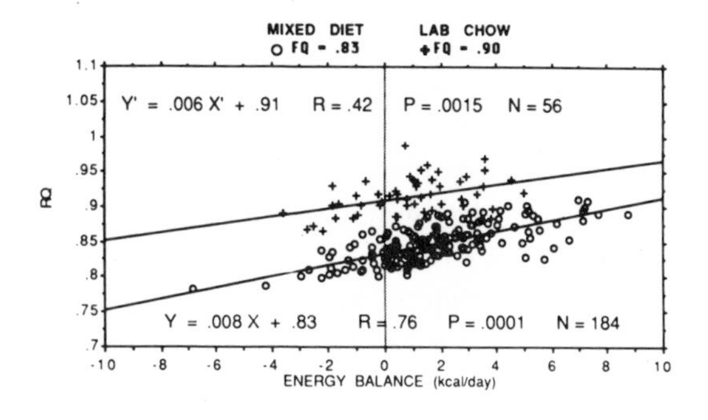

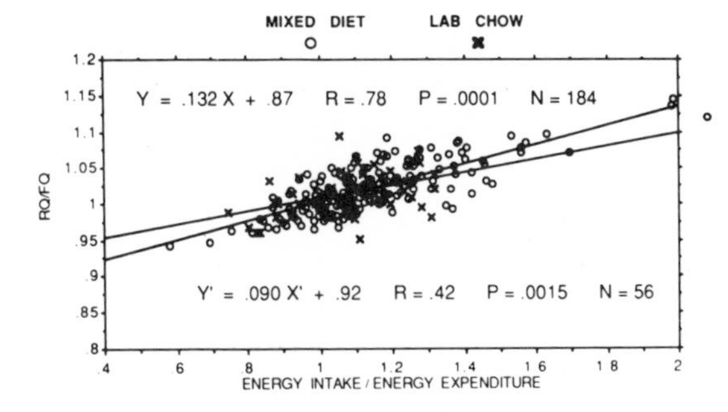

Fig. 7. Relationship between RQ/FQ ratios and daily energy balances in *ad libitum* fed mice. For experimental conditions, see legend to Fig. 1.

metabolic regulatory phenomena exist, but it is important to realize that changes in the operating range of the body's glycogen reserves and in its adipose tissue mass contribute also to the achievement of this condition. The fat-to-carbohydrate ratio of the diet is therefore a factor in determining for which body composition the steady-state of weight maintenance will be achieved. Failure of appropriately reducing the range within which glycogen levels are maintained on diets with a substantial fat content will require an expansion of the adipose tissue mass, to raise FFA levels and to enhance fat oxidation until it is commensurate with the proportion of fat in the diet. Maintenance of glycogen reserves below the level of saturation is made less likely by the high palatibility and ubiquitous availability of foods. Thus one should expect a high incidence of obesity in affluent societies consuming mixed diet with a relatively high fat content, particularly when physical activity is too limited to substantially enhance the oxidation of fat relative to that of glucose.

In metabolic terms, the goal of weight maintenance resides in the achievement of an average RQ equal to the FQ of the diet (or lower if a lesser body weight is to be achieved). This is easier when a diet with a reduced fat content is selected, because its FQ is relatively high. Additional leverage is provided by aerobic exercise, owing to its effect in decreasing the RQ.

Acknowledgments

This work was supported by NIH grant DK33214. The collaboration of K.E.G. Sargent and B.R. Krauss is gratefully acknowledged.

REFERENCES

1. Flatt, J.P. (1978). The biochemistry of energy expenditure. *In "Recent Advances in Obesity Research,"* Bray, G.A., ed., Vol. 2, pp. 211-228. Newman, Washington, D.C.
2. Flatt, J.P. (1987). Dietary fat, carbohydrate balance, and weight maintenance; effects of exercise. *Am. J. Clin. Nutr.* **45**, 296-306.
3. Flatt, J.P. (1987). The difference in the storage capacities for carbohydrate and for fat, and its implications in the regulation of body weight. *N. Y. Acad. Sci.* **499**, 104-123.
4. Acheson, K.J., Schutz, Y., Bessard, T., Ravussin, E., Jéquier, E., and Flatt, J.P. (1984). Nutritional influences on lipogenesis and thermogenesis after a carbohydrate meal. *Am. J. Physiol.* **246**, E62-E70.
5. Flatt, J.P., Ravussin, E., Acheson, K.J., and Jéquier, E. (1985). Effects of dietary fat on post-prandial substrate oxidation and on carbohydrate and fat balances. *J. Clin. Invest.* **76**, 1019-1024.
6. Bjorntorp, P., Bergman, H., Varnauskas, E., and Lindholm, B. (1969). Lipid mobilization in relation to body composition. *Metabolism* **18**, 841-851.
7. Golay, A., Felber, J.P., Meyer, H.U., Curchod, B., Maeder, E., and Jéquier, E. (1984). Study of lipid metabolism in obesity diabetes. *Metabolism* **33**, 111-116.
8. Christensen, E.H. and Hansen, O. (1939). Arbeitsfahigkeit und Ernahrung. *Skand. Arch. Physiol.* **81**, 160-171.
9. Bielinski, R., Schutz, Y., and Jéquier, E. (1985). Energy metabolism during the post-exercise recovery in man. *Am. J. Clin. Nutr.* **42**, 69-82.

Diet and Obesity, Bray, G.A. et al., eds., pp. 205–217.
Japan Sci. Soc. Press, Tokyo/S. Karger, Basel (1988)

Dieting Using a Very Low Calorie Diet

SATORU TSUKAHARA, MAKOTO OHNO, AND
YOSHIO IKEDA

*Third Department of Internal Medicine, Jikei University
School of Medicine, Tokyo 105, Japan*

Obesity is frequently accompanied by diabetes mellitus and many other diseases whose prevention or treatment may require a weight reduction. Appropriate diet therapy and exercise ought normally to lead to smooth weight reduction, but in clinical practice many difficulties are experienced, and despite the especially great need for rapid weight reduction in morbid obesity, the body weight of such individuals has been difficult to reduce (*1*).

Much attention has been attracted to very low calorie diet (VLCD) which limits daily energy intake to less than 500 kcal in obese patients. The therapeutic principle of VLCD is to provide no more high-quality protein than needed to prevent degradation of lean body mass (LBM) and no more carbohydrates than needed to prevent severe ketosis, while satisfying vitamin and mineral requirements. Such a diet prevents the occurrence of severe adverse effects while achieving a comparable weight reduction to that attained by starvation therapy.

However, considerable interindividual variations exist in the degree of LBM loss caused by VLCD, and not all the metabolic

TABLE I
Characteristics of Study Groups

	VLCD	
	240 kcal/day	420 kcal/day
Number of subjects	11	13
Male	3	5
Female	8	8
Age (yrs)	34±12	34±16
Weight (kg)	79.5±14.3	87.3±21.5
% IBW	160.0±29.2	157.0±22.4

effects of VLCD have been elucidated (*2*). The purpose of this review is to present our experimental findings and to discuss the effects of VLCD on weight reduction and on the protein metabolism of the human body.

I. STUDY PROTOCOL

The clinical features of subjects are shown in Table I. The subjects were 24 moderately obese patients; nine were simple obesity without any complications, eight had diabetes mellitus, and seven had impaired glucose tolerance (IGT) according to WHO criteria of 75 g oral glucose tolerance test (OGTT). Eleven patients received VLCD of 240 kcal per day for 4 weeks and 13 patients were treated by VLCD of 420 kcal per day. Three out of 11 in the first group were male and eight were female; five of the thirteen in the second group were male and eight were female. The average age in both groups was 34 years. The two groups' average % ideal body weight (IBW) was also well matched: 160% and 157%. The % IBW was calculated by modified Broca method.

The screening examination consisted of medical history, physical examination, blood pressure, chest and abdominal X-rays, electrocardiogram, urinalysis, blood cell count, blood chemistry including transaminase, electrolyte, blood urea nitrogen, uric acid, lipid, and plasma glucose measurements. Based on the screening test, patients with serious diseases other than diabetes mellitus, hyperlipidemia, and hyperuricemia were eliminated. Eighteen of the 24 subjects were inpatients, six were outpatients. In both cases, for at least 3 weeks before the initiation of VLCD, the patients' dietary intake was restricted to 23–30 kcal/kg IBW. VLCD was introduced when the rate of weight reduction from the previous regimen began to decline.

All subjects received one each of the two VLCD. The formula diets used in the study were Modifast® and Optifast®, consisting of processed egg albumin in powder form. The three packs of Modifast® provide a daily energy intake of 240 kcal, 33 g of protein, 25.5 g of carbohydrate, and 0.7 g of fat. The five packs of Optifast® provide a daily energy intake of 420 kcal, 70 g of protein, 30 g of carbohydrate, and 2.0 g of fat. Both formula diets contain sufficient amount of vitamins and minerals. They are mixed with 200 ml of cold or warm water, and patients are required to drink at least 2 l of water during a day. Exercise was limited to daily activities and patients were advised to avoid strenuous exertion.

The patients were weighed daily. The nitrogen balance was measured three times a week. Serum concentrations of transferrin, prealbumin (PA), and retinol-binding protein (RBP), representative rapid turnover proteins were determined twice a week by the radial immunodiffusion method (*3*). The plasma concentrations of amino acids were analyzed once a week by high performance liquid chromatography method (*4*). Nitrogen balance was calculated from excreted amounts of urinary urea nitrogen. Non-urinary nitrogen excretion was uniformly assumed to be 2 g per day.

During VLCD, blood cell count, blood chemistry, electrolyte blood pressure, electrocardiogram, urinalysis, and blood gas analysis were repeatedly performed to guarantee the patients' safety.

II. WEIGHT LOSS

The changes in weight at the end of each week during the 4 weeks of VLCD are shown in Fig. 1. On the 240 diet, the average patient's weight decreased from 79.5 kg to 71.2 kg. On the 420 diet, it declined from 87.3 kg to 79.4 kg. The average weight reduction

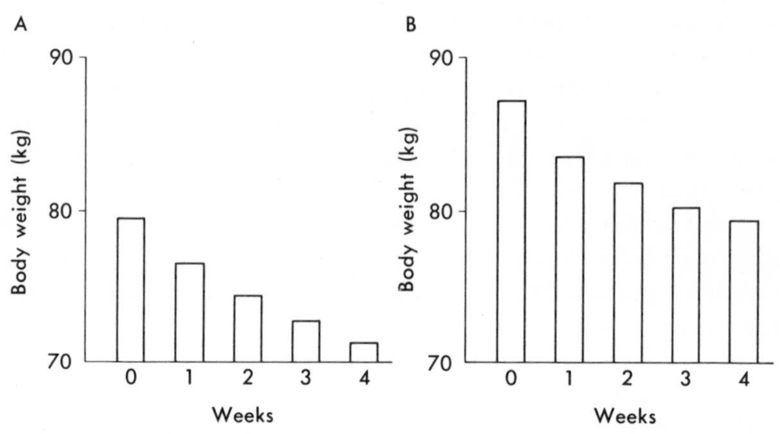

Fig. 1. Weight loss during 4 weeks of VLCD. A: 240 kcal/day. B: 420 kcal/day.

was 8.3 ± 1.7 kg in the 240 diet group and 7.9 ± 2.0 kg in the 420 diet group. No significant difference was obtained between the weight reducing effects of the two regimens. In both cases, the weight reduction tended to be greatest during the first week and to diminish gradually thereafter. Other investigators reported the same weight reducing effect (7–10 kg) in a short term treatment of 4 weeks (*5*) and about 20 kg weight reduction in a treatment of 3 months (*6*).

III. NITROGEN BALANCE

The changes in average nitrogen balance in 10 patients on the 240 diet are shown in Fig. 2. The tendency to have negative balance gradually improved after the first week, but it was still present at the end of the 4 weeks of VLCD. Five out of 10 patients recovered a positive nitrogen balance, while five still tended to have a negative one.

On the other hand, the negative nitrogen balance was less severe in the 420 diet than in the 240 diet, and by the end of the fourth week the average nitrogen balance recovered positive in the 420 diet (Fig. 3). Five out of 7 patients recovered a positive balance, while

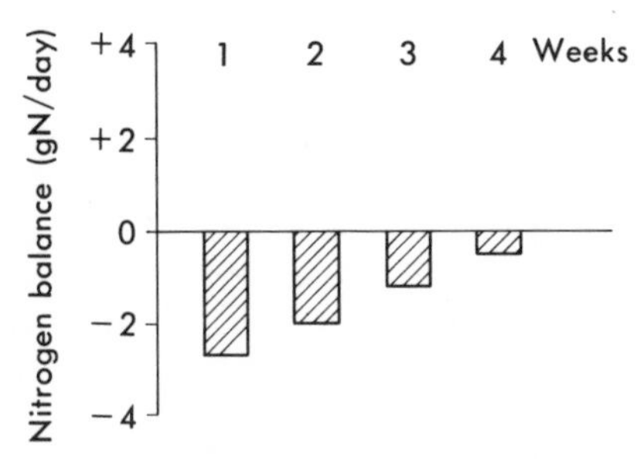

Fig. 2. Average daily nitrogen balance at different weeks during VLCD of 240 kcal/day.

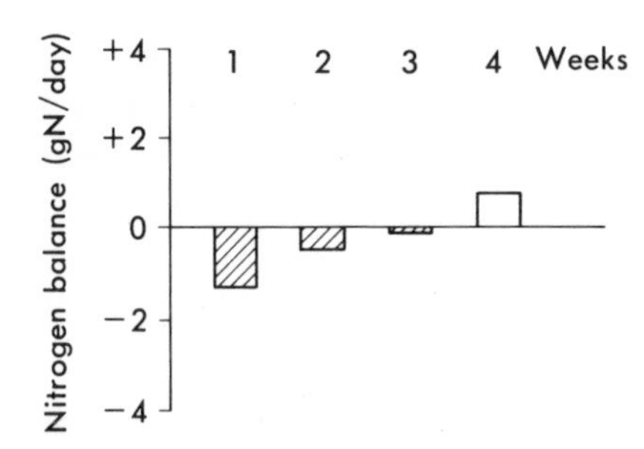

Fig. 3. Average daily nitrogen balance at different weeks during VLCD of 420 kcal/day.

two were still negative at the end of the study. This indicates that a better nitrogen balance is achieved with VLCD of 420 kcal, which provides 70 g of protein. In other words, 70 g of protein corresponds to 1.0 g to 1.5 g protein per kg IBW in Japanese.

The protein requirement with VLCD has been discussed. Howard and MacLean-Baired (*7*) studied the nitrogen balance on VLCD of 260 kcal, containing 25 g of egg albumin and 40 g of carbohydrate. In their study, the nitrogen balance was achieved at the end of 4 weeks on VLCD. The faecal and cutaneous nitrogen losses were extremely small, therefore, they concluded that the non-urinary nitrogen loss could be ignored in the calculation of nitrogen balance. Hoffer *et al.* (*8*) examined the nitrogen balance of

TABLE II
Changes in Serum Proteins on VLCD

	VLCD	Day 0	Day 14	Day 28
Albumin	240 kcal/day	4.4±0.4	4.5±0.2	4.3±0.3
(mg/dl)	420 kcal/day	4.7±0.4	4.7±0.1	4.4±0.4
Transferrin	240 kcal/day	259.6±15.5	265.4±36.1	228.3±29.0
(mg/dl)	420 kcal/day	261.3±98.7	259.3±42.2	230.2±45.4
PA (mg/dl)	240 kcal/day	31.4±7.2	22.2±4.2*	20.7±5.5**
	420 kcal/day	38.5±10.8	29.5±7.7*	26.4±11.9*
RBP (mg/dl)	240 kcal/day	4.6±1.6	3.2±1.7**	2.7±0.7**
	420 kcal/day	4.3±1.2	3.4±1.0**	2.9±1.2**

*$p<0.05$, **$p<0.01$.

two different VLCD of 500 kcal. One diet provided 1.5 g protein/kg IBW; the other provided 0.8 g protein/kg IBW plus 0.7 g carbohydrate/kg IBW. They showed that the nitrogen balance was achieved at 3 weeks on a diet of 1.5 g high quality protein/kg IBW when non-urinary nitrogen excretion was taken into account.

However, Fisler *et al.* (*9*) reported that 10 obese males were still negative in nitrogen balance at the end of 3 weeks when consuming a diet of 1.3 g protein per kg IBW. They found that only four of 10 subjects were able to attain positive nitrogen balance after 5 weeks, but other subjects continued negative balance after 8 weeks. Yang *et al.* (*10*) also showed the difference in ability to attain nitrogen balance between obese subjects consuming a sufficient amount of protein. In our study, there was observed an individual variation in their ability to conserve body nitrogen. Further studies are needed to clarify these variabilities in nitrogen conservation during VLCD.

IV. RAPID TURNOVER PROTEIN

Table II shows the changes in serum albumin, transferrin, PA, and RBP before and the second and the fourth weeks after the initiation of VLCD. Levels of serum albumin concentration hardly changed. Levels of serum transferrin concentration tended to decrease without statistical significance; in none of the individual

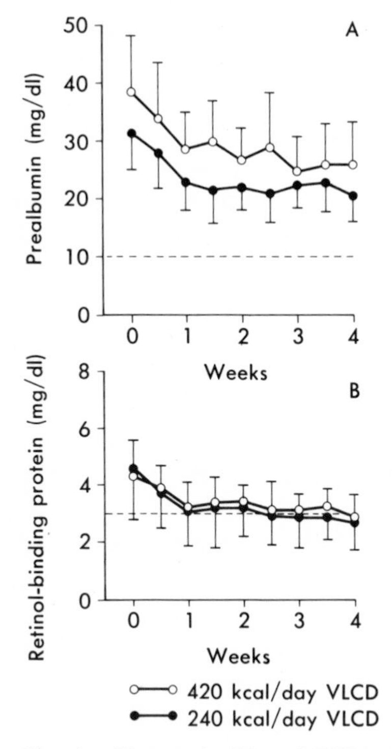

Fig. 4. Changes in PA and RBP on VLCD.

cases did the level fall below the lower limit of normal range.

As shown in Fig. 4, levels of serum PA and RBP began to fall immediately after the initiation of VLCD and continued to decrease slowly even after the first week. Levels of both PA and RBP fell significantly on both the 240 diet and the 420 diet.

Values for serum PA stayed within the normal range in all patients throughout VLCD of 4 weeks. In the case of serum RBP, however, the average level fell below the lower limit of normal range 2 to 3 weeks after the initiation of the 240 diet and did not return to the normal level during the 4-week study. In patients on the 420 diet, the average level of serum RBP fell below the lower limit of normal range after 4 weeks.

Plasma proteins, albumin, transferrin, PA, and RBP have been used to assess protein-calorie malnutrition (*11*). Subclinical malnutrition was encountered in hospitalized patients and also in obese subjects on low calorie diets. There is no doubt that the low concentration of albumin reflects severe protein-calorie malnutrition; however, its half-life is about 20 days, and a large extravascular pool exists. Therefore, serum albumin is not a sensitive indicator for nutritional assessment of dietary deprivation for short-term periods.

Transferrin is a carrier protein of iron and plays an important role in hemoglobin synthesis and iron metabolism. Evaluation of serum transferrin in nutritional assessment was shown by Reeds (*12*) and Blackburn *et al.* (*13*). Its half-life is 7 to 10 days, shorter than that of albumin. On the other hand, when serum transferrin synthesis is elevated in iron deficiency anemia, its usefulness in nutritional assessment becomes less sensitive (*14*).

Two serum proteins, PA and RBP are synthesized in the liver, and are called rapid turnover proteins. Serum concentrations of these two rapid turnover proteins are much smaller, and each has a short half-life (PA: 2 days, RBP: 10–20 hr). Shetty *et al.* (*15*) studied the effect of protein and energy restriction on these plasma proteins in 16 obese women. They concluded that PA and RBP were more sensitive indices for dietary restriction than was either albumin or transferrin.

A few studies were performed to ascertain the factors which correlate with nitrogen balance. Only Fisler *et al.* (*9*) have shown the significant relationship between total nitrogen loss and decreasing serum levels of complement C_3. In our study, the correlation between total nitrogen loss, calculating nitrogen excretion for 4 weeks, and the decreasing serum levels of rapid turnover protein was analyzed. A positive correlation was observed between total nitrogen loss and $\varDelta$PA (Fig. 5). A trend to correlate between total nitrogen loss and $\varDelta$RBP was observed but without statistical significance (Fig. 5). Thus we found that serum prealbumin measurement is an effective indicator for the degradation of LBM when consuming VLCD.

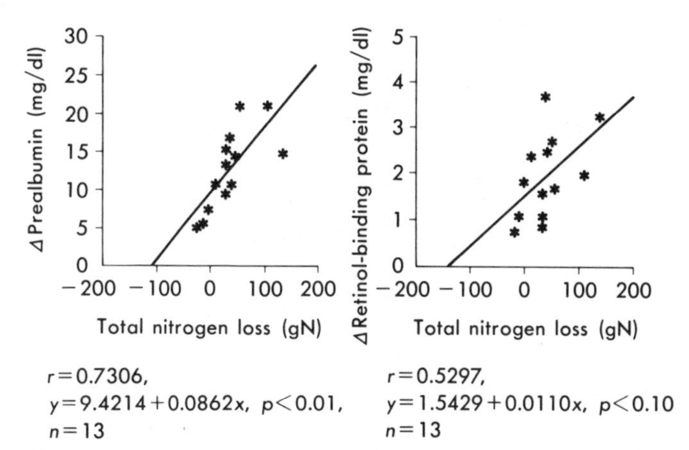

Fig. 5 Correlation between total nitrogen loss and ⊿PA, ⊿RBP.

V. AMINO ACID

The weekly average concentrations of branched chain amino acids were measured in 8 out of 13 patients consuming the 420 diet. Plasma valine, leucine, and isoleucine levels increased transiently after the first week, but then gradually decreased, and by the end of the study they returned very close to the basal levels (Fig. 6).

Figure 7 shows changes in plasma glucogenic amino acids. Plasma levels of glutamic acid, alanine and threonine tended to decrease slowly. Plasma histidine decreased significantly.

The changes in plasma levels of tyrosine, phenylalanine, and tryptophan are shown in Fig. 8. Levels of all three substances decreased. The decrease in the plasma phenylalanine level was significant ($p<0.05$), and the concentration of plasma tryptophan also decreased significantly ($p<0.01$).

Plasma branched chain amino acids increased transiently and glucogenic amino acids decreased, suggesting that a part of the energy requirements is supplied from amino acids which are derived from the breakdown of muscle protein during VLCD.

Average total essential amino acids fell from 955 μM/l to 821 μM/l and average total nonessential amino acids fell from 2,294

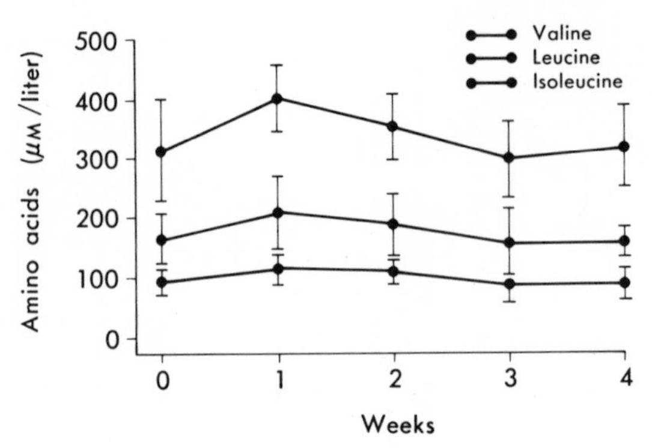

Fig. 6. Plasma concentration of branched-chain amino acids during VLCD.

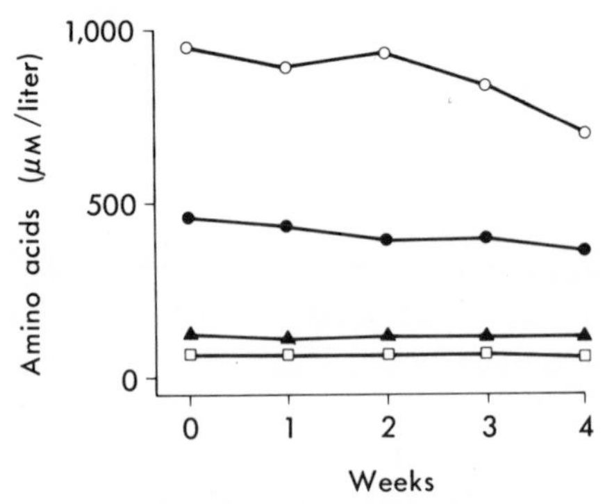

Fig. 7. Plasma concentration of glucogenic amino acids during VLCD. ○ glutamic acid; ● alanine; ▲ threonine; □ histidine.

μM/l to 1,938 μM/l. However, the ratio of essential to nonessential amino acids hardly changed: 0.416 to 0.424. Judging from this ratio, no severe nutritional disorders occurred with this VLCD regimen.

Plasma amino acid concentrations are, however, important determinants of intracellular protein synthesis and degradation. It is well known that branched chain amimo acids, in particular, play an important role in the regulation of protein metabolism (*16*). In this study, the branched chain amino acids returned to nearly basal levels after 4 weeks, when the positive nitrogen balance was achieved

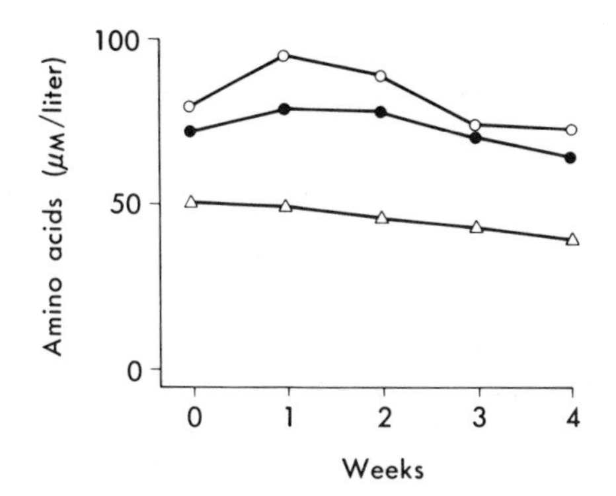

Fig. 8. Plasma concentration of amino acids during VLCD. ○ tyrosine; ● phenylalanine; △ tryptophan.

in VLCD of 420 kcal. Since the branched chain amino acids are relatively easily influenced by catabolism, the changes in their plasma levels may be considered to reflect the degree of catabolism. Hence, the altered LBM and transition in branched chain amino acids appear to be closely interrelated.

SUMMARY

To evaluate the effect of two different VLCD by observing weight reduction and nitrogen conservation, 11 obese subjects received 240 kcal per day (P33 g, C25.5 g), and 13 other obese subjects were treated by using 420 kcal per day (P70 g, C30 g). The VLCD of 420 kcal showed an almost identical effect on weight reduction as that attained by VLCD of 240 kcal. The VLCD of 420 kcal showed smaller loss of LBM than the other by providing a sufficient amount of protein. A positive correlation was observed between total nitrogen loss and the decreasing levels of serum prealbumin concentration.

Thus we concluded that serum prealbumin measurement was an effective indicator for the degradation of LBM when consuming VLCD. Branched chain amino acids increased transiently and some glucogenic amino acids decreased, thereby revealing gluconeogenesis from muscle protein during consumption of VLCD. The ideal VLCD regimen for obese Japanese is approximately 400 kcal per day, providing 60 g protein and 40 g carbohydrate.

REFERENCES

1. Stunkard, A.J. and McLaren-Hume, M. (1959). The results of treatment for obesity. *Arch. Intern. Med.* **103**, 79–85.
2. Wadden, T.A., Stunkard, A.J., and Brownell, K.D. (1983). Very low calorie diets: their efficacy, safety, and future. *Ann. Intern. Med.* **99**, 675–684.
3. Mancinni, G., Carbonara, A.O., and Heremans, J.F. (1965). Immunological quantitation of antigens by single radial immunodiffusion. *Immunochemistry* **2**, 235–254.
4. Lee, P.L.Y. (1974). Single-column system for accelerated amino acid analysis of physiological fluids using five lithium buffers. *Biochem. Med.* **10**, 107–121.
5. Howard, A.N., Grant, A., Edwards, O., Littlewood, E.R., and McLean-Baired, I. (1978). The treatment of obesity with a very-low-calorie liquid-formula diet: an inpatient/outpatient comparison using skimmed milk as the chief protein source. *Int. J. Obesity* **2**, 321–332.
6. Tuck, M.L., Sowers, J., Dornfeld, L., Kledzik, G., and Maxwell, M. (1981). The effect of weight reduction on blood pressure, plasma renin activity, and plasma aldosterone levels in obese patients. *N. Engl. J. Med.* **304**, 930–933.
7. Howard, A.N. and MacLean-Baired, I. (1977). A long-term evaluation of very low calorie semi-synthetic diets; and inpatient/outpatient study with egg albumin as the protein source. *Int. J. Obesity* **1**, 63–78.
8. Hoffer, L.J., Bistrian, B.R., Young, V.R., Blackburn, G.L., and Matthews, D.E. (1984). Metabolic effects of very low calorie weight reduction diets. *J. Clin. Invest.* **73**, 750–758.
9. Fisler, J.S., Drenick, E.J., Blumfield, D.E., and Swendseid, M.E. (1982). Nitrogen economy during very low calorie reducing diets: quality and quantity of dietary restriction. *Am. J. Clin. Nutr.* **35**, 471–486.
10. Yang, M-N., Barbosa-Saldivar, J.L., Pi-sunyer, F.X., and Van Itallie, T.B. (1981). Metabolic effects of substituting carbohydrate for protein in a low calorie diet: a prolonged study in obese outpatients. *Int. J. Obesity* **5**, 231–236.
11. Young, G.A. and Hill, G.L. (1978). Assessment of protein calorie malnutrition in surgical patients from plasma proteins and anthropometric measurements. *Am. J. Clin. Nutr.* **31**, 429–435.
12. Reeds, P.J. (1976). Serum albumin and transferrin in protein-energy malnutrition and the prognosis of severe undernutrition. *Br. J. Nutr.* **36**, 255–263.
13. Blackburn, G.L., Bistrian, B.R., Maini, B.S., Schlamm, H.T., and Smith, M.F. (1977). Nutritional and metabolic assessment of the hospitalized patient. *J.*

Parent. Ent. Nutr. **1**, 11-22.
14. Delpeuch, F., Cornu, A., and Chevalier, P. (1980). The effect of iron deficiency anemia on two indices of nutritional status, prealbumin and transferrin. *Br. J. Nutr.* **43**, 375-379.
15. Shetty, P.S., Watrasiewiez, K.E., Jung, R.T., and James, W.P.T. (1979). Rapid-turnover transport proteins: an index of subclinical protein malnutrition. *Lancet* **ii**, 2310-2312.
16. Adibi, S.A. (1980). Roles of branched chain amino acids in metabolic regulation. *J. Lab. Clin. Med.* **95**, 475-484.

Diet and Obesity, Bray, G.A. et al., eds., pp. 219–227.
Japan Sci. Soc. Press, Tokyo/S. Karger, Basel (1988)

Effect of Capsaicin on Body Fat Deposition

SHUICHI KIMURA AND CHIHO LEE

Laboratory of Nutrition, Department of Food Chemistry, Tohoku University, Sendai 980, Japan

Taste perception is one of the most important factors in food discrimination because recognition and acceptance of food mainly depends on its chemostimulatory characteristics. In addition, the organism's nutritional state brought about by food acts as a metabolic signal to the regulatory centers and modulates oral responses to food (*1, 2*). The relationship between taste preference and nutritional state is, therefore, an important area of investigation.

In this series of studies we found that the appetite or preference for sodium chloride depends not only on genetic factors but also on the nutritional status, *i.e.*, dietary protein levels (*3*). We also observed that consumption of "umami," especially monosodium glutamate, had a reducing effect on sodium chloride intake (*4*). This phenomenon suggests that the preference for salty taste was modified by certain condiments. Thus, capsaicin (CAP) appeared in this study.

Capsaicin and its derivatives are the pungent components of hot red pepper, which came from Mexico originally and is now used all over the world as a condiment. The chemical formula is shown

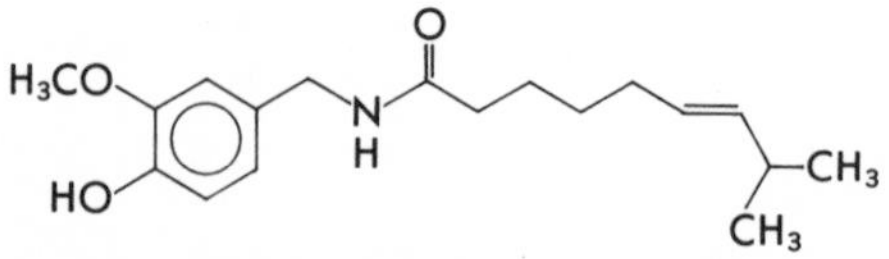

Fig. 1. Structure of CAP.

in Fig. 1.

Iwai and his coworkers have demonstrated that CAP is readily transported through the gastrointestinal tract and is absorbed *via* a non-active transport system into the portal vein; most absorbed CAP is then excreted as metabolites *via* the urine within 48 hr in rats (*5*).

Recently they also observed that CAP enhances energy metabolism and stimulates catecholamine secretion from the adrenal medulla (*6*).

The present study was conducted in two major phases: first, effect of CAP on taste preference for sodium chloride and, second, effect of CAP on body fat deposition.

I. TASTE PREFERENCE STUDIES USING RATS

As experimental animals, Okamoto and Aoki's spontaneously hypertensive rats (SHR) and Wistar-slc rats were used and they were divided into groups according to dietary protein levels, 5% (low) and 15% (high) purified whole egg protein diet groups; these two groups were further divided into two groups, with and without CAP. Capsaicin was supplemented as 0.014% of the diet by weight. The percentage of CAP used in this study was approximately that usually ingested by people living in rural Thailand (*7*). The animals were allowed free choice of deionized water containing 0, 0.5, 0.9, and 1.4% sodium chloride as drinking water (Fig. 2). After an 8-week feeding period, rats were sacrificed. Liver triglyceride was extracted by the method of Folch *et al.* (*8*). The levels of triglyceride in plasma and liver were measured by the enzymatic method of glycerol-3-phosphate oxidase using an assay kit (Wako Pure Chemical Industries, Ltd., Osaka), and the level of phospholipid in plasma

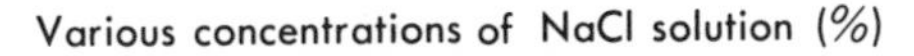

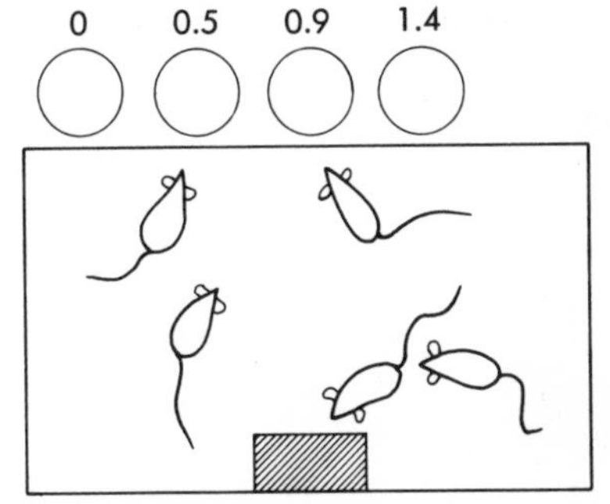

Fig. 2. The design of the preference test in rats.

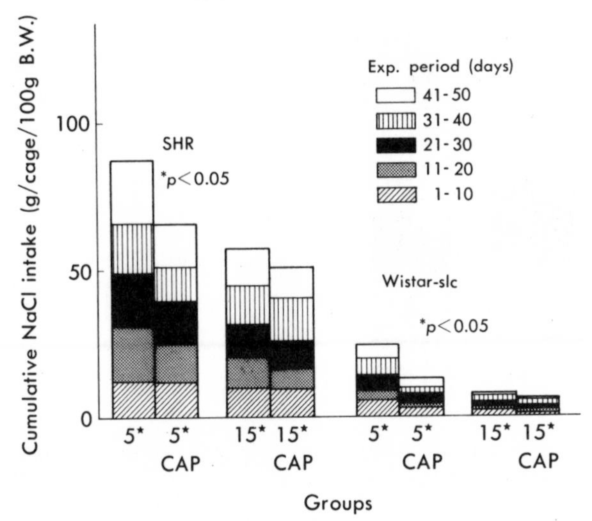

Fig. 3. The effect of CAP and dietary protein levels on the cumulative NaCl intake. *Dietary protein level.

was also measured by the enzymatic method of choline oxidase-peroxidase using as assay kit (Wako Pure Chemical Industries, Ltd., Osaka).

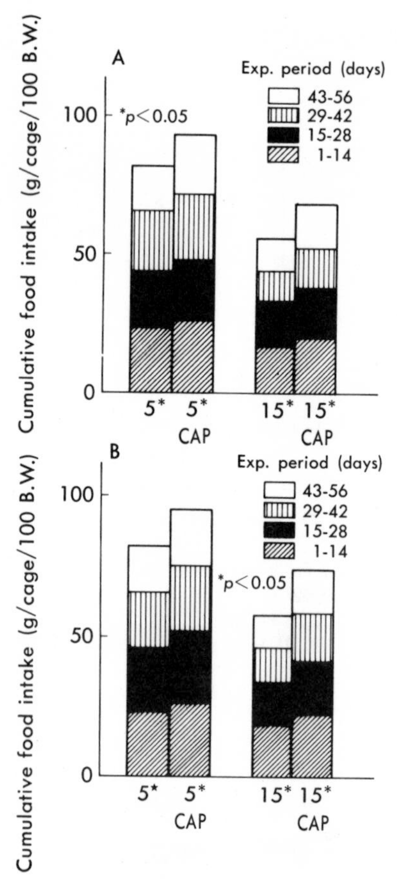

Fig. 4. The effect of CAP and dietary protein levels on the cumulative food intake by SHR (A) and Wistar-slc (B) rats.

II. EFFECT OF CAPSAICIN ON TASTE PREFERENCE FOR SODIUM CHLORIDE

In SHR for both low and high-dietary protein levels, the most acceptable sodium chloride concentration was 0.9%, as shown previously (*4*). Rats fed the low protein diet showed a preference not only for the 0.9% solution but also more concentrated sodium

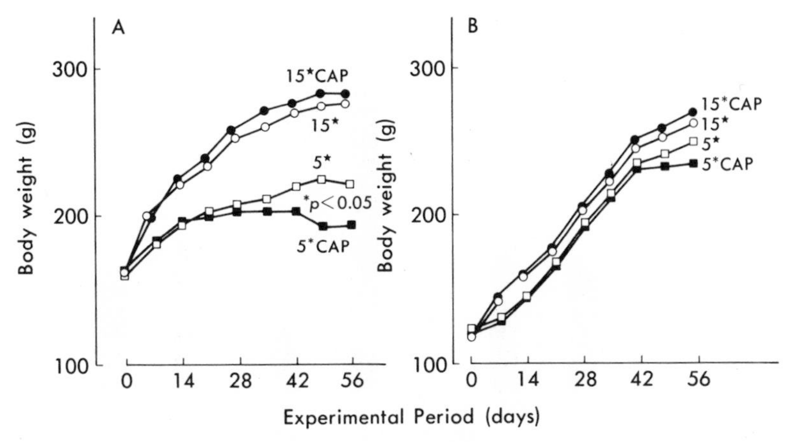

Fig. 5. The effect of CAP and dietary protein levels on the weight gain in SHR (A) and Wistar-slc (B) rats. *Dietary protein level.

chloride solutions (1.4%). The cumulative amount of sodium chloride ingested by SHR fed the low protein diet was clearly higher than that of SHR given the high protein diet, and it was found that CAP had a definite reducing effect on the consumption of sodium chloride in this preference test (Fig. 3). This tendency was also observed in Wistar-slc rats although they generally preferred deionized water.

The result of this experiment demonstrated that CAP has a reducing effect on sodium chloride intake.

III. EFFECTS OF CAPSAICIN ON THE BODY FAT DEPOSITION

The general tendency for a stimulative effect by CAP on food intake was observed in all experimental groups, and significant differences were recognized between with and without CAP in low protein·SHR and high protein·Wistar-slc groups (Fig. 4). However, food intake did not always reflect body weight gain as shown in Fig. 5, and, in fact, significantly less body weight gain was observed in the low protein·Wistar-slc group. In a low protein diet-condition, the weight of perirenal adipose tissue of rats fed CAP was signi-

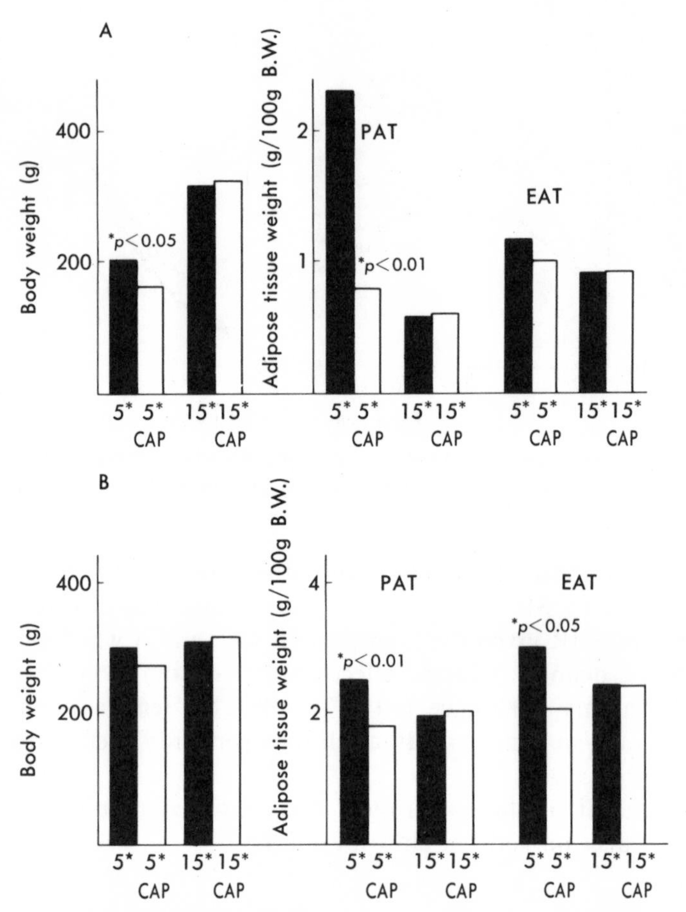

Fig. 6. The effect of CAP and dietary protein level on body weight and adipose tissue weight. A: SHR rats. B: Wistar-slc rats. *Dietary protein level. PAT, perirenal adipose tissue; EAT, epididymal adipose tissue.

ficantly less than that of non-supplemented rats in both SHR and Wistar-slc (Fig. 6). On the other hand, the weight of epididymal adipose tissue of rats fed CAP was also significantly less than that of non-supplemented Wistar-slc rats. These results suggest that CAP may stimulate energy consumption, and also that it might be effective in repressing fat deposition.

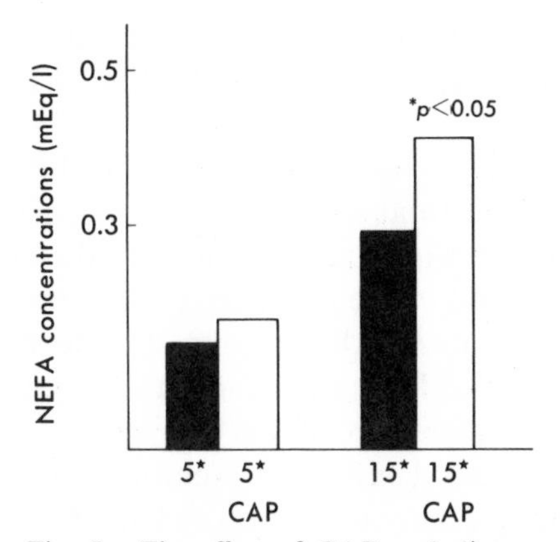

Fig. 7. The effect of CAP and dietary protein levels of serum NEFA in Wistar-slc rats.

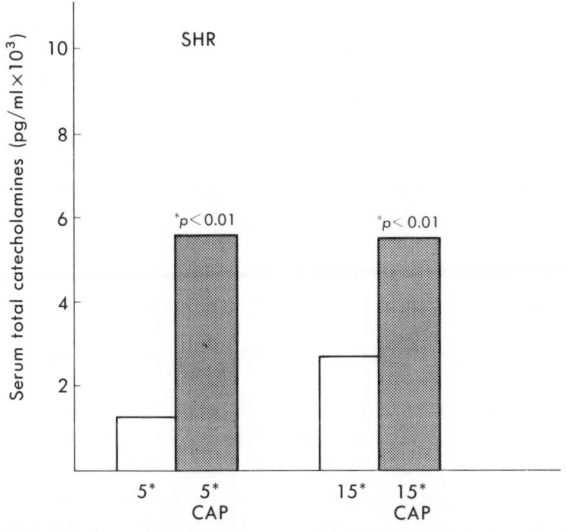

Fig. 8. The effect of CAP and dietary protein levels of serum catecholamines in SHR.

In 1975 Fregly reported that SHR constitutionally has a large appetite for salt (*9*). This may be the animal's genetic nature. However, our previous studies and present results suggested strongly that the taste preference for salt depends not only on genetic factors but also on the nutritional status, and some condiments have modification-effects.

Condiments generally have a stimulatory action on the appetite; in fact, CAP stimulates food intake by rats. However, another biological activity of this material may act to stimulate the energy consumption. Recently, Iwai and his coworkers (*10*) have been increasing the facts known about CAP. In our studies it was observed that levels of nonesterified fatty acids and catecholamine in plasma were elevated with the ingestion of CAP (Figs. 7 and 8). Capsaicin may thus be a useful foodstuff for preventing obesity. In general, condiments have unique characteristics and their components are complicated. It is well known that some of the physiological effects depend on nutritional state of the organism. Therefore, establishment of an individual methodology might be important in the use of CAP to prevent obesity.

SUMMARY

Capsaicin stimulates food intake but represses sodium chloride intake and fat accumulation in rats. The effect of CAP on body fat accumulation is greater in the lower protein diet.

REFERENCES

1. Boudreau, J.C. (1980). Taste and the taste of foods. *Naturwissenschaften* **67**, 14-20.
2. Bertoin, M., Beauchamp, G.K., and Engelman, K. (1982). Long-term reduction in dietary sodium alters the taste of salt. *Am. J. Clin. Nutr.* **36**, 1134-1144.
3. Kimura, S., Yokomukai, Y., and Komai, M. (1987). Salt consumption and nutritional state especially dietary protein level. *Am. J. Clin. Nutr.* **45**, 1271-1276.
4. Kimura, S., Yokomukai, Y., and Komai, M. (1987). Effects of dietary protein level and Umami on taste preference for sodium chloride. *In* "A Umami: A Basic Taste," Kawamura, Y. and Kare, M.R., eds., pp. 611-634. Marcel Dekker, New York and Basel.
5. Kawada, T. and Iwai, K. (1985). *In vivo* and *in vitro* metabolism of dihydrocapsaicin, a principle of hot pepper, in rat. *Agric. Biol. Chem.* **49**, 441-448.
6. Watanabe, T., Kawada, T., and Iwai, K. (1987). Enhancement by capsaicin of

energy metabolism in rats through secretion of catecholamine from adrenal medulla. *Agric. Biol. Chem.* **51**, 75-79.

7. Interdepartment Comittee on Nutrition for National Defense (1962). Nutrition survey—the kingdom of Thailand, pp. 57-59. U.S. Government Printing Office, Washington, D.C.
8. Folch, T., Lees, M., and Sloane-Stanley, G.H. (1957). A simple method for the isolation and purification of total lipids from animal tissues. *J. Biol. Chem.* **226**, 497-509.
9. Fregly, M.J. (1975). NaCl intake and preference threshold of spontaneously hypertensive rats. *Proc. Soc. Exp. Biol. Med.,* **149**, 915-920.
10. Watanabe, T., Kawada, T., Yamamoto, M., and Iwai, K. (1987). Capsaicin, a pungent principle of hot red pepper, evokes catecholamine secretion from the adrenal medulla of anesthetized rats. *Biochem. Biophys. Res. Commun.* **142**, 259-264.

PERSPECTIVE

Future Research in Obesity

GEORGE A. BRAY

Department of Medicine, University of Southern California, Los Angeles, CA 90033, U.S.A.

My assignment has been to review possible future directions for research to solve important problems relating to obesity and its health implications. To accomplish this task, I will first review the information available in 1977 and the progress we have made in the past 10 years in four major areas. These will be: 1) improvements in our techiques for estimating body composition; 2) the epidemiologic base on which health risks associated with obesity can be estimated; 3) improved understanding of the mechanisms which control food intake, metabolism of fat cells and energy expenditure; and 4) treatments for obesity. In each of these four areas, the status in 1977 will be briefly summarized and the additional information developed over the next 10 years presented in outline form. This will be followed by some recent studies from our laboratory on the modification of regional fat distribution. We will ask the question, "Can regional fat distribution be modulated?" and will summarize three recent studies from our laboratory on this question. Finally, a summary of future directions will be proposed based on recent developments.

I. IMPROVED TECHNIQUES FOR MEASURING BODY COMPOSITION

In 1977 a variety of techniques were available for estimating body dimensions and the body composition (Table I).

The most widely used of these techniques are still of great use and are based on anthropometry, including measurements of height and weight, skinfold thickness, body circumferences and body breadths. Beginning with the work of Behnke and Wilmore (*1*), the technique of density measurement for estimating body fat came into wide use and was the 'gold standard' for measuring body composition in the past 40 years (*2*). Various chemical, radioactive and non-radioactive isotopes have also been used for estimating various body compartments for more than 10 years (*3–5*). Total body water can be estimated from the dilution of antipyrine as well as from tritiated water (^3H_2O) or deuterium oxide (D_2O). Body fat can be directly estimated from dilution xenon or cyclopropane. The final major technique available for measuring body composition in 1977 was the use of the naturally occurring isotope of potassium (^{40}K).

During the last 10 years a number of new and sophisticated techniques have been added to the armamentarium which allow not only quantitation of fat and non-fat components in the body but also accurate estimate of their regional distribution. The first of these is the measurement of impedance or body conductivity (*6*). The total body electrical conductivity system has been developed for grading meat in terms of fat content and has been recently applied to the measurement of body fat in human beings. The expense of this instrument, however, will limit its current usefulness. A simple technique for estimating body impedance may see more widespread

TABLE I
Obesity-body Composition

1977	1987
Anthropometry	Bioelectric impedance
Density	Computed tomography
Isotope dilution	Magnetic resonance images
Ultrasound	Neutron activation

use if formulas can be developed for reliably estimating fat from this technique which involves attaching electrodes to an arm and leg and measuring the intermediate impedance. The computed tomography can be used to give estimates of subcutaneous and intra-abdominal fat and has been applied for this purpose by several laboratories (*7*). Even more elegant pictures contrasting subcutaneous and intra-abdominal fat can be obtained by magnetic resonance imaging (MRI). In these pictures the fat depots stand out as white compared to the tissues which contain water and other components (*8*). Finally, a total body neutron activation allows estimates not only of total composition of water and fat but also of calcium, protein, and other components. Utilizing these techniques our ability to quantitate total fat and estimate its regional distribution has been markedly improved during the past decade.

II. THE EPIDMIOLOGIC BASE FOR ESTIMATING THE RISKS OF OBESITY

In contrast with the elegant laboratory techniques which have become available for estimating body fatness and its distribution, the application of these techniques to population studies lags far behind. In 1977 there were several important studies available from which concerns about obesity and health were estimated (Table II).

These included several life insurance studies (*9*), the 18-year follow-up of the Framingham Study (*10*), the seven country study of Keys and his collaborators (*11*) and the Pooling project (*12*). The life insurance studies have consistently suggested that increased body weight was associated with higher mortality and that the major causes of this excess risk were heart disease, digestive diseases, and diabetes.

Several prospective studies, however, suggested that obesity was not an independent risk factor for mortality but rather that obesity might have its effects through its association with hypertension or with diabetes. Data from long term follow-up studies from Canadian Air Force pilots in the Manitoba project (*13*) and for younger individuals in the Los Angeles civil servants study suggested that a

TABLE II
Estimating Risks for Obesity

1977	1987
Build and Blood Pressure 1959	Build Study 1980
Health Examination Survey 1961–1963	National Health Examination Surveys, 1971–1974; 1976–1980
Framingham Study 18 years	Framingham Study-30 years
Ten State Nutrition Survey	American Cancer Society Study
Cross-town Manhattan Study	Scandanavian Studies

different picture might emerge with newer data.

Over the past 10 years several new studies have appeared which have solidified our understanding of the relationships of weight and obesity to health. The Build Study of 1979 (*14*) from the life insurance industry confirmed their earlier findings. The Framingham data at 26 and 30 years (*15, 16*) indicated a similar relationship between weight and mortality as estimated in the life insurance studies, with a minimum mortality rate associated with an entry body mass index of 22 for all age groups. In addition, the 26-year follow-up indicated that obesity was an important predictor of risk of heart attacks, particularly among women. The American Cancer Study with its 750,000 people also demonstrated the important relationship between increasing body mass and the risks for heart disease, diabetes mellitus, and digestive diseases (*17*). This study also made clear that certain forms of cancer, particularly those of the uterus, ovary, and breast in women and prostate and colon in men also showed a small but significant increase, particularly in the very heavy groups. Finally, two Scandanavian studies have added to our knowledge base. The large population base study in Norway showed the similarity of mortality for under and overweight individuals of both sexes at all ages confirming the relationship in previous studies (*18*). Finally, the studies in Gothenberg (*19, 20*) and in Milwaukee (*21*) demonstrated the important relationship between abdominal fat and risk for diabetes, hypertension, stroke, cardiovascular disease, and overall mortality. Indeed, recognition of the importance of increased abdominal fat for all of the risks associated with obesity provides one of the important advances of the past decade and focuses on key questions which need answering in the years ahead.

III. MECHANISMS FOR POSITIVE FAT BALANCE

Development of obesity implies deposition of increased amounts of fat or alternatively a positive fat balance. Understanding the processes by which this occurs has been steady, but less dramatic than our understanding of the relative risks described above.

In 1977 the statement "calories do count" would have been widely accepted. The anatomic basis for considering the problem of obesity focused on the dual center hypothesis with the ventromedial satiety and lateral feeding centers (*22*). The principal neurotransmitters were considered to be monoaminergic and to involve norepinephrine and dopamine (Table III).

In the past decade our focus has shifted from the dual center hypothesis with two anatomic nuclei to a dual control mechanism

TABLE III
Mechanisms for Obesity

1977	1987
Food intake	
Calories do count	Hyperphagia NOT essential
Dual center hypothesis	Autonomic hypothesis
Monoamine neurotransmitters	Peptide neurotransmitters
Fat cells	
Hyperplastic obesity	Hyperplasia after puberty
Fat cells fixed at puberty	Alpha-2 inhibitory and beta-stimulatory receptors
Beta-receptor and lipolysis	Lipoprotein lipase as gatekeeper
	Adipsin
Thermogenesis	
Basal RMR related to surface area	RMR is familial
TEF NOT different in obese	Sympathetic component in TEF
Luxusconsumption present	Sodium pump, brown fat and futile cycles implicated in obesity

involving in important ways the control of the autonomic nervous system (*23*). Thus those conditions associated with reduced body fat (lateral hypothalamic lesions) appear to have increased sympathetic activity and those with increased body fat (ventromedial hypothalamic lesions) genetic obesity to have reduced activity of the sympathetic nervous system (*24*).

The role of calories has also changed. It is now apparent that most experimental types of obesity can develop in the absence of increased quantity of food intake (*24*). The most striking and complex development in the area of food intake has come from the recognition that numerous peptides found in the gastrointestinal tract are also found in the brain and that many of these have important effects on food intake. Three groups of endogenous opioid peptides have been identified and characterized during the past decade, and two of them can stimulate feeding. Similarly, two peptides from the family of pancreatic polypeptides are also known to stimulate food intake when injected to the paraventricular nucleus (*25*).

On the other hand, several peptides have been identified which have potent inhibitory effects on food intake. These include cholecystokinin, calcitonin, and corticotrophin releasing factor (CRF) (*26*). CRF is of particular interest because adrenalectomy has been demonstrated to reverse weight gain or its progression in essentially all forms of experimental obesity (*24*). Since CRF increases in the brain and presumably in the cerebral spinal fluid of animals following adrenalectomy, this peptide may play an important role in this process.

Finally, in addition to the ventromedial and lateral hypothalamic areas, it has become clear that the paraventricular nucleus with its rich supply of peptides is also important in the regulation of food intake. Modulating this system are not only the monoamines norepinephrine and epinephrine, but also clearly serotonin. As will be noted below, drugs related to the metabolism of serotonin have become agents in the treatment of obesity because any agent which enhances serotonin or serotonin-like effects is associated with a reduction in body weight.

In 1977 Hirsch and his colleagues (*27*) along with Bjorntorp and his associates (*28*) had clearly identified the hyperplastic and hypertrophic types of obesity. Moreover, it was dogma at that time that the hyperplastic type of obesity developed in childhood and that by the end of puberty, the number of fat cells was fixed.

It had also become clear by 1977 that in human beings, adipose tissue triglyceride stores arose primarily from fatty acids obtained from circulating lipoproteins and that lipoprotein lipase (LPL) thus played a crucial role in the entry of fatty acids from circulating triglycerides into the adipose tissue pool of fatty acids (*29*).

Over the past decade our views about the time in which multiplication of new fat cells ends has changed. In experimental animals it is now clear that the number of cells of animals in some fat deposits can increase after the end of the pubertal growth spurt (*30*). There is also data in human beings suggesting that increasing fat stores in adult life may also be associated with an increase in the number of fat cells (*7*). Knowledge about the mechanisms controlling lipolysis have increased substantially. The beta receptor mediated activation of adenylate cyclase with the formulation of cAMP was already known in 1977 (*31*). However, it has become clear that there is an important alpha-2 adrenergic inhibitory system operative in human fat cells and that this alpha-2 adrenergic inhibitory system varies from one fat deposit to another (*32*). It now appears that the major differences associated with regional fat deposits relate to the density of the alpha-2 adrenergic receptors on human fat cells.

It has also been demonstrated that LPL, the so-called gatekeeper for fat storage by fat cells, remains high following weight loss (*33*) whereas most other abnormal parameters of obesity tend to return to normal. Some have suggested that this activity of LPL may play an important role in the tendency to regain weight after weight loss.

In 1977 the relationship of energy expenditure to body surface area, body weight and fat free mass had been clearly demonstrated (*3, 4*). Based on the work of Sims and his colleagues (*34*) as well as that of Miller and associates in London (*35, 36*), the concept of individual differences in response to excess energy intake, categorized as those who gain weight easily and those who gain weight with difficulty (luxusconsumption), has reemerged from a period where this concept was thought to have succumbed (*37*). Mechanisms for this effect were poorly understood and it provided one of the fascinating developments of the past decade (*38*).

Studies on weight gain during overfeeding have demonstrated important genetic components in this process (*39*). Not only are genetic components demonstrated in the process of ease or difficulty of weight gain, but also in the familial association of resting energy expenditure within families (*40*). Studies on the mechanisms for differences have suggested a role for the sympathetic nervous system, which is activated during intravenous infusion of glucose and insulin (*41*). It has been shown that part of the increased oxygen consumption produced by infusing glucose and insulin can be blocked by administration of a beta adrenergic blocking drug (*42*). This suggests that there are beta receptors which mediate energy expenditure related to glucose disposal. Changes in energy efficiency during weight gain and weight loss have sparked renewed interest in the question of whether weight cycling, that is, gaining and losing and regaining weight, may be more hazardous than maintaining a stable weight (*43*).

IV. TREATMENT OF OBESITY

In 1977 a number of treatments were used for obese patients. Diet and exercise were the standard recommendations, with new varieties of dietary advice being published each year to captivate the gullible. Behavior modification was already in wide use. Pioneering studies with this approach were first published in 1967 and the ensuing 10 years had seen the practical application of these ideas become widely disseminated. It was clear even then that programs which incorporated behavior modification techniques had improved short and long term results.

Starvation or the zero calorie diet was waning in popularity. Introduced in 1959, it had spread widely as a way of getting weight off quickly in the hospital. Problems such as hypotension, kidney

TABLE IV
Treatments of Obesity

1977	1987
Diet and exercise	Diet and exercise
Behavior modification	Behavior modification
Starvation	Very low calorie diets
Appetite suppressants	Appetite suppressants
Thyroid hormone	Serotonin-like drugs
Jejuno-ileal bypass	Thermogenic drugs
	Jaw-wiring
	Vagotomy
	Gastric restriction

stones, loss of protein, and poor long term results led to the introduction of diets with only small amounts of protein. Gradually these evolved into the very low calorie diets, sometimes mistakenly called protein-sparing modified fasts. The past 10 years has seen an explosion in the use of these diets, both under medical supervision and without. It would appear desirable to have very low calorie diets medical supervision.

The early 1970's saw the release by the Food and Drug Administration of three new appetite suppressants which were derivatives of amphetamine. Due to abuse and addiction to amphetamine, all drugs in this group received a bad name with a resultant decrease in their usage. Although there are many trials with these drugs, the use of a good behavioral program can do as well as the drugs in many instances (*44, 45*). With the recognition that serotonin played an important role in reducing food intake (*46*) and that thermogenic mechanisms were important in regulating body weight (*38*), new approaches to drug therapy were developed. Trial drugs for both of these mechanisms are now being tested.

The surgical approaches to obesity have evolved rapidly. Jejuno-ileal bypass, an operation which connected the first 35 cm or so of jejunum to the terminal 10 cm of ileum, was in wide use in 1977. By the end of the decade, however, it had been largely replaced by gastric restrictive operations. The metabolic and inflammatory consequences of J-I bypass were unacceptable. In contrast, the

TABLE V
Recommendations for Next Decade

1. Study mechanisms for local fat deposition and for this effect on health.
2. Examine basis for interaction of peptides and monoamines in control of single meals *versus* long term regulation of fat.
3. Identify genetic markers for obesity and the environmental system with which they act.
4. Develop improved methods of treatment.

number of complications associated with gastric restriction has been less. Weight loss, however, may not be as good. Jaw-wiring is less invasive than gastric surgery but less effective in the long run. One major use of jaw-wiring has been as a technique of rapid weight loss prior to a gastric operation. Vagotomy has been given a trial in treatment of obesity but has not received wide use. Surgical treatment is palliative. For massively obese individuals, it may be the best we currently have to offer, but it is still only palliative.

V. RECOMMENDATIONS

From this review of advances in our knowledge over the past 10 years, several conclusions and recommendations are possible. First, regional fat distribution, particularly the deposition of fat in the abdominal and probably the intra-abdominal region, is a far more important health hazard than a comparable increase in fat in other regions. The important questions remaining to be answered are whether intra and extra abdominal subcutaneous fat are equally important and why fat accumulates in one region as opposed to another. One possible clue to this mechanism is the data of Evans and Kissebah (*47*), who have shown a correlation between free testosterone and upper or abdominal fat. The mechanisms by which testosterone is increased in some women and the differential effects in men are questions of utmost importance.

A second area of considerable importance is our understanding of food intake. In clinical treatment protocols there appears to be a maximal weight loss of about 10 kg, even with prolonged treatment.

This suggests that there must be redundancy in the control mechanisms for fat stores and raises the possibility that effective treatment of obesity may require more than a single approach. Additional information about the regulation of food intake and its role in the development of obesity will certainly come from enhanced understanding of the mechanisms by which adrenalectomy reverses or prevents the development of experimental types of obesity. Clarifying the role of the centrally acting peptides in feeding may also have important clinical dividends. A third area of considerable importance is the role of genetic and environmental interaction in individuals who gain weight easily. Understanding of the mechanisms for familial aggregation of energy expenditure may provide important clues to the cellular mechanisms by which these genetic factors are manifested and thus to the potential differences in risk for developing obesity. Finally, treatments for obesity are woefully inadequate. Recent data suggests that weight cycling, the so-called rhythm method of girth control or the yo-yo syndrome may be hazardous to one's health. This needs to be clearly documented. Newer approaches to the therapy of obesity, particularly the abdominal type of obesity, are of importance because of the risks which individuals with this type of fat distribution have for the development of diabetes, hypertension, stroke, and heart attack. In conclusion, I would suggest that the past decade has seen great strides and that we are standing on the threshold of an exciting era in the understanding of obesity and the approaches for its effective treatment of disorders of positive fat balance.

SUMMARY

During the past 10 years a number of important advances have been made in the study of obesity. Measurement of body composition has improved through the introduction of techniques for determining total body electrical conductivity, body impedance computerized tomography and neutron magnetic resonance. With these techniques both regional fat and total body fat can be estimated with great accuracy. Reduced energy expenditure has been shown to be predictive of the risk of gaining weight. In addition, a variety of neurointestinal peptides have been shown to stimulate or inhibit feeding. New treatments for obesity in the past 10 years include drugs which enhance thermogenesis and drugs which can raise the concentration of serotonin in the central nervous system. Gastric operations have replaced jejuno-ileal bypass as the major surgical treatment for obesity. Blockade of adrenergic receptors by topical treatment has been shown to reduce localized fat deposits. These advances over the past decade offer great promise for treatment of obesity in the years ahead.

REFERENCES

1. Behnke, A.R. and Wilmore, J.H. (1974). "Evaluation of Body Build and Composition." Prentice-Hall, Englewood Cliffs.
2. Lohman, T.G. (1981). Skinfolds and body density and their relation to body fatness: A review. *Hum. Biol.* **53**, 181–225.
3. Bray, G.A. (1976). "The Obese Patient: Major Problems in Internal Medicine," pp. 1–450. Saunders, Philadelphia.
4. Garrow, J.S. (1978). "Energy Balance and Obesity in Man," 2nd Ed. Elsevier, New York.
5. Moore, F.D., Olesen, K.H., McMurrey, J.D., Parker, H.V., Ball, M.R., and Boyden, C.M. (1963). "The Body Cell Mass and Its Supporting Environment in Body Composition in Health and Disease," p. 23. Saunders, Philadelphia.
6. Segal, K.R., Gutin, B., Presta, E., Wang, J., and Van Itallie, T.B. (1985). Estimation of human body composition by electrical impedance methods: A comparative study. *J. Appl. Physiol.* **58**, 1565–1571.
7. Sjostrom, L. and William-Olsson, T. (1981). Prospective studies on adipose tissue development in man. *Int. J. Obesity* **5**, 597–604.
8. Cohn, S.H., Vartsky, D., Yasamura, S., Sawitsky, A., Zanzi, I., Vaswani, A., and Ellis, K.J. (1980). Compartmental body composition based on total-body nitrogen, potassium, and calcium. *Endocrinol. Metab.* **2**, E524–E530.
9. Society of Actuaries (1959). Build and blood pressure study. Society of Actuaries, Chicago.
10. Kannel, W.B. and Gordon, T. (1979). Physiological and medical concomitants of obesity: The Framingham Study. *In* "Obesity in America," Bray, G.A., ed., DHEW Publication No. (NIH) 79–359, pp. 125–153. U.S. Government Printing Office, Washington, D.C.
11. Keys, A., Menotti, A., Aravanis, C., Blackburn, H., Djordevic B.S., Buzina, R., Dontas, A.S., Fidanza, F., Karvonen, M.J., Kimura, N., Mohacek, I., Nedelj-

kovic, S., Puddu, V., Punsar, S., Taylor, H.L., Conti, S., Kromhout, D., and Toshima, H. (1984). The seven countries study: 2,289 deaths in 15 years. *Prev. Med.* **13**, 141-154.
12. The Pooling Project Research Group (1978). Relationship of blood pressure, serum cholesterol, smoking habit, relative weight and ECG abnormalities to incidences of major coronary events: Final report of the Pooling Project. *J. Chron. Dis.* **31**, 201-306.
13. Rabkin, S.W. Mathewson, F.A., and Hsu, P.H. (1977). Relation of body weight to development of ischemic heart disease in a cohort of young North American men after a 26-year observation period: The Manitoba Study. *Am. J. Cardiol.* **39**, 452-458.
14. Society of Actuaries (1979). Build Study of 1979. Society of Actuaries and Association of Life Insurance Medical Directors of America.
15. Feinleib, M. (1985). Epidemiology of obesity in relation to health hazards. *Ann. Intern. Med.* **106**, 1019-1024.
16. Hubert, H.B., Feinleib, N., McNamara, P.M., and Castelli, W.P. (1983). Obesity as an independent risk factor for cardiovascular disease: A 26-year follow-up of participants in the Framingham Heart Study. *Circulation* **67**, 968-977.
17. Lew, E.A. and Garfinkel, L. (1979). Variations in mortality by weight among 750,000 men and women. *J. Chron. Dis.* **32**, 563-576.
18. Waaler, H.T. (1983). Height, weight and mortality: The Norwegian experience. *Acta. Med. Scand.* **679**, 1-55.
19. Lapidus, T., Bengtsson, L.C., Larsson, B., Pennert, K., Rybo, E., and Sjostrom, L. (1984). Distribution of adipose tissue and risk of cardiovascular disease and death: A 12 year follow-up of participants in the population study of women in Gothenburg, Sweden. *Br. Med. J.* **289**, 1257-1261.
20. Larsson, B., Svardsudd, K., Welin, L., Wilhelmsen, L., Bjorntorp, P., and Tibblin, G. (1984). Abdominal adipose tissue distribution, obesity, and risk of cardiovascular disease and death: 13 year follow-up of participants in the study of men born in 1913. *Br. Med. J.* **288**, 1401-1404.
21. Kissebah. A.H., Vydelingum, N., Murray, N., Evans., D.J., Hartz, D.J., Kalkoff, R.K., and Adams, P.W. (1982). Relation of body fat distribution to metabolic consequences of obesity. *J. Clin. Endocrinol. Metab.* **54**, 254-260.
22. Bray, G.A. and York, D.A. (1971). Genetically transmitted obesity in rodents. *Physiol. Rev.* **51**, 598-646.
23. Bray, G.A. and York, D.A. (1979). Hypothalamic and genetic obesity in experimental animals: An autonomic and endocrine hypothesis. *Physiol. Rev.* **59**, 719-809.
24. Bray, G.A. (1987). Obesity—A disease of nutrient or energy balance? *Nutr. Rev.* **45**(2), 33-43.
25. Leibowitz, S. (1986). Brain monoamines and peptides: Role in the control of eating behavior. *Fed. Proc.* **45**, 1396-1403.
26. Morley, J.E. and Levine, A.S. (1985). The pharmacology of eating behavior.

Annu. Rev. Pharmacol. Toxicol. **25**, 127–146.
27. Hirsch, J. and Batchelor, B. (1976). Adipose tissue cellularity in human obesity. *Clin. Endocrinol. Metab.* **5**, 299–311.
28. Bjorntorp, P. (1974). Effects of age, sex, and clinical conditions on adipose tissue cellularity in man. *Metabolism* **11**, 1091–1102.
29. Greenwood, M.R.C. (1985). Adipose tissue: Cellular morphology and development. *Ann. Intern. Med.* **103**, 996–999.
30. Faust, I.M., Johnson, P.R., Stern, J.S., and Hirsch, J. (1978). Diet-induced adipocyte number increase in adult rats: A new model of obesity. *Am. J. Physiol.* **235**, E279–E286.
31. Burns, T.W., Langley, P.E., Terry, B.E., Bylund, D.B., Hoffman, B.B., Tharp, M. D., Lefkowitz, R.J., Garcia-Saintz, J.A., and Fain, J.N. (1981). Pharmacological characterizations of adrenergic receptors in human adipocytes. *J. Clin. Invest.* **67**, 467–475.
32. Lafontan, M., Dang-Tran, L., and Berlan, M. (1979). Alpha adrenergic antilipolytic effect of adrenaline in human fat cells of the thigh. Comparison with adrenaline responsiveness of different fat deposits. *Eur. J. Clin. Invest.* **9**, 261–266.
33. Schwartz, R.S. and Brunzell, J.D. (1981). Increase of adipose tissue lipoprotein lipase activity with weight loss. *J. Clin. Invest.* **67**, 1425–1430.
34. Sims, E.A.H. (1986). Energy balance in human beings: The problems of plenitude. *Vit. Horm.* **43**, 1–43.
35. Miller, D.S. and Mumford, P. (1967). Gluttony. I. An experimental study of overeating low- or high-protein diets. *Am. J. Clin. Nutr.* **20**, 1212–1222.
36. Miller, D.S., Mumford, P., and Stock, N.J. (1967). Gluttony. II. Thermogenesis in overeating man. *Am. J. Clin. Nutr.* **20**, 1223–1229.
37. Newburgh, L.H. (1944). Obesity: I. Energy metabolism. *Physiol. Rev.* **24**, 18–31.
38. Rothwell, N.J. and Stock, M.J. (1981). Regulation of energy balance. *Annu. Rev.* **1**, 235–256.
39. Bouchard, C. (1985). Body composition in adopted and biological siblings. *Hum. Biol.* **57**, 61–75.
40. Bogardus, C., Lillioja, S., Ravussin, E., Abbot, W., Zawadzski, J.K., Young, A., Knowler, W.C., Jacobowitz, R., and Moll, P.P. (1986). Familial dependence on the resting metabolic rate. *N. Engl. J. Med.* **315**, 96–100.
41. Ravussin, E., Bogardus, C., Schwartz, R.S., Robbins, D.C., Wolfe, R.R., Horton, E.S., Danforth, E., Jr, and Sims, E.H. (1983). Thermic effect of infused glucose and insulin in man. Decreased response with increased insulin resistance in obesity and noninsulin-dependent diabetes mellitus. *J. Clin. Invest.* **72**, 893–902.
42. Acheson, K., Jequier, E., and Wahren, J. (1983). Influence of B-adrenergic blockade on glucose-induced thermogenesis in man. *J. Clin. Invest.* **72**, 981–986.
43. Brownell, K.D. (1982). Obesity: Understanding and treating a serious, prevalent, and refractory disorder. *J. Consult. Clin. Psychol.* **50**, 820–840.
44. Stunkard, A.J., Wilcox, O.N., Craighead, L., and O'Brien, R. (1980). Controlled trial of behaviour therapy, pharmacotheraphy, and their combination in the

treatment of obesity. *Lancet* **ii**, 1045–1047.

45. Dahms, W.T., Molitch, M.E., Bray, G.A., Greenway, F.L., Atkinson, R.L., and Hamilton, K. (1978). Treatment of obesity: Cost-benefit assessment of behavioral therapy, placebo, and two anorectic drugs. *Am. J. Clin. Nutr.* **3**, 774–778.
46. Blundell, J.E. (1984). Serotonin and appetite. *Neuropharmacology* **23**, 1537–1552.
47. Evans, D.J., Hoffman, R.K., Kalkhoff, R.K., and Kissebah, A.H. (1983). Relationship of androgenic activity to fat topography, fat cell morphology, and metabolic aberrations in premenopausal women. *J. Clin. Endocrinol. Metab.* **57**, 304.

Subject Index